The Birthkeepers

Reclaiming an ancient tradition

Veronika Sophia Robinson
Illustrated by Andri Thwaites

The Birthkeepers: reclaiming an ancient tradition
© 2008 Veronika Sophia Robinson
ISBN 978-0-9560344-1-0

Published by Starflower Press
www.starflowerpress.com

Cover illustration of Isis by Andri Thwaites
Illustrations by Andri Thwaites

Also by the same author:
The Drinks Are On Me: everything your mother never told you about breastfeeding (illustrated by Andri Thwaites)
The Compassionate Years ~ a history of the RSPCA in New Zealand
Field of Lavender (poetry)
Howl at the Moon (contributing poet) published by Wild Women Press

British Library Cataloguing in Publication Data.
A catalogue record for this book is available from the British Library.

Author's note: midwives are referred to in the feminine form as either she or her. This is done for no other reason than for ease of reading, as compared to s/he or his/her.

The author's notes can be found in the back of the book. She has deliberately avoided the traditional use of unsightly numerical footnotes.

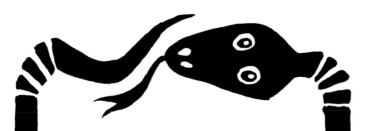

Interior artwork:

The illustrations used throughout this book are captured within the essence of the snake. I was born and grew up in Australia, and spent my childhood being 'dead scared' of snakes. We lived rurally, and they were part of the landscape, so to speak. Through my esoteric and metaphysical studies, I have come to see the snake in a new way, despite my primitive reflex to run like the wind when I come across one slithering through the grass.

A snake symbolises 'sloughing off'. The snake sheds its old skin to make way for the new, and acts as a shamanic teacher, representing deep-level transformation of the psyche, and opens us to Creation's amazing mysteries.

In order for women to become Birthkeepers of the ancient tradition, they need to slough off old ideas and identities which hold them prisoner to the dominant birth culture.

Cover illustration:

Isis is the Goddess of fertility and motherhood, and female Creator in history and mythology. Isis means female of the throne.

The Greeks adopted her as Sophia, which means Divine Wisdom. She is an appropriate choice for the Birthkeepers theme.

Dedicated, with grace, to three wise women:

My mother ~ Angelikah ~ who brought eight babies Earthside, and her three youngest boys into this world free of medical observation and supervision. I owe my beautiful mother so very much, for it is she who taught me, in her wise, quiet way, to think outside the boxes of nutrition, birth and spirituality, and into authentic living, and being true to one's self. Thank you mum, for being my friend. This book's seed came from you.

Author of Unassisted Childbirth ~ Laura Kaplan Shanley ~ a leading light in the field of unassisted childbirth. Thank you for being a friend and inspiration. We first 'met' when my midwife gave me a copy of your book, after realising I wanted total freedom in my birth experience. The respect and admiration I have for you, Laura, have greatly increased over the years. You're beautiful, radiant and incredibly passionate. This book grew because of you.

The late, great Jeannine Parvati Baker ~ friend and peer ~ arrived Earthside June 1, 1949, and returned to her Breathmaker on December 1, 2005. Her life was well-lived, as a lay midwife, ashtanga yogini, astrologer, founder of Hygieia College, herbal medicine-woman, mother of six, author of Prenatal Yoga & Natural Childbirth, Hygieia: A Woman's Herbal, and co-author, with Rico Baker, of Conscious Conception.

She coined the terms Birthkeeper, Freebirth and Paid Paranoid. The world owes an enormous amount of gratitude to her visionary, pioneering ways in reclaiming family as the central focus of society. The title of this book is a namesake to your life's work, Jeannine ~ a fellow 12th house denizen. It was you who taught me that the stellium in the 12th house of my natal chart means that my life path equates to "serve or suffer". This book blossomed for you.

Part One ~ The Labour

Part Two ~ The Birth
The Birthkeepers speak

Part Three
Third stage

See no light
Hear no talk
Allow no eyes
~ Mantra of a wise birthing wombyn

Introduction

My mother had her last three children at home, unassisted. She'd merely wanted a homebirth, but her doctor was too afraid to attend. What to do? Well, she chose to give birth to her children without him. Kamahl was born in the bathroom. René arrived in her bedroom on my dad's birthday. The cord was around his neck, but my mother calmly removed it. It was not a moment for fear, or for ringing an ambulance. Albert was born in the bathroom. For her, it was a test of faith: a test in the Divine.

I suppose, for me, it was this normal and natural approach to birth that allowed me to see Freebirth for what it is, rather than what the media and most birth professionals suggest. I've known babies die or be brain-injured in medically-managed births, but thankfully, I have never heard, first hand, of death due to a consciously planned unassisted birth.

Since the beginning of The Mother magazine, women have called me for advice and support on their unassisted birthing journeys. I've always reminded them that the power was with them, not me or anyone else. I merely acted to remind them that they had everything within them they needed to birth their babies beautifully and gently into this world.

What we see is a reflection
of who we are,
where we are at
on our life's journey,
and what we believe.
Birth is our mirror.

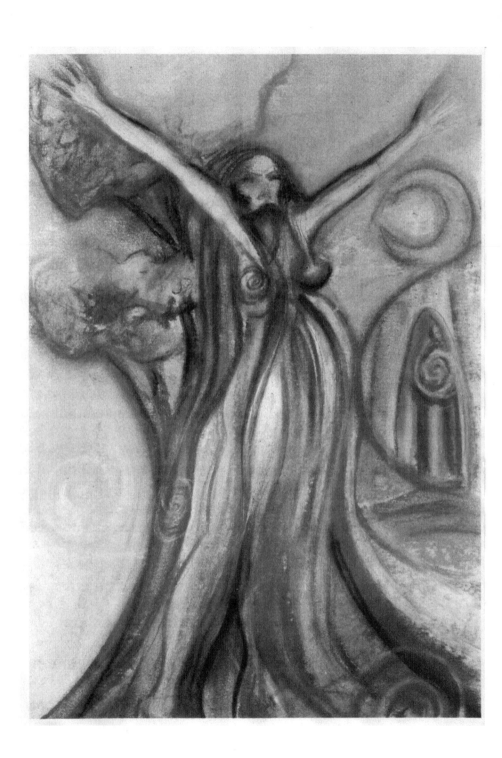

Our birth is but a sleep and a forgetting:
the soul that rises with us,
our life's Star,
hath had elsewhere its setting,
and cometh from afar:
not in entire forgetfulness,
and not in utter nakedness,
but trailing clouds of glory do we come,
From God, who is our home.

~ William Wordsworth

Thank you

My deepest gratitude goes to The Birthkeepers, near and far, seen and unseen. Thank you too, to the gorgeous wombyn whose stories fill these pages: Fabienne; Clara; Julie; Kate; Julia; Amelia; Cath; Clio; Zeynep; Sara; Mara and Ornella. Jeannine Parvati Baker, for encouraging us to know that by healing birth we could heal the Earth. She coined the term Birthkeeper as a marriage of Earthkeeper and Birth.

An Earthkeeper is a Native American word for eco-activist, as well as a holder of sacred, Earth-based wisdom. I chose the title of this book in gratitude to Jeannine for all that she was, and all that she did for mothers, fathers and children everywhere.

Andri Thwaites, my friend, and visionary artist, for once again honouring me by illustrating, with love, passion, vision and belief, according to the pictures in my head, for which I had no way of extracting myself. You are my artistic angel. Thank you.

My daughters, Bethany Angelika and Eliza Serena: thank you to both of you for teaching me about the yin and yang of birth ~ both humbling me, and exalting me. Mostly, for opening me wide, wide, wide.

My mother, Angelikah, for giving me a copy of Leboyer's Birth Without Violence, during my formative years. You knew it would touch me deeply.

My soul's love, and husband through this lifetime's journey, Paul, for birthing our babies with me; for knowing when to whisper, touch, laugh, hold me all night long; and when to sing our children lullabies.

Karen Arnott, web mistress, for making beautiful public spaces to promote my work, and seamlessly translating techno-stuff. Simon Marston, master of all things technical, for never complaining about my computer and technical phobias and illiteracy.

And last, but never least, my ancestresses ~ for all the tears you bring to my eyes, both in sadness and in joy. I wear your birth stories in my veins, and your power and strength in my heart. Let me never forget your journeys. *Namaste, Veronika*

Foreword

My hope is that I can encourage men and women to re-vision birth: to see it as a physical manifestation of their deepest beliefs, fears and desires. My dream is to share the beauty and simplicity of birth ~ as nature intended ~ and mirror to women and their partners the courage to create a birth which amplifies the Universal messages of love, peace, gratitude and kindness.

I have the deepest desire to see every baby born in a space of love, reverence and holiness, in recognition of both their sentience and their Divinity, physical and spiritual; and for their parents to recognise both the sanctity and everydayness of such a miraculous and momentous occasion, and to prepare for the moment as consciously as possible. For some people, this will take the form of an unassisted childbirth (Freebirth). My intention is that the messages in this book be utilised by all birthing families, regardless of whether they plan an unobserved birth at home, or birth in a hospital, or any of the variations in-between. I hope to take the mystery out of childbirth by explaining, in the simplest terms, why some women birth majestically and easily, and why others scream out as if in torture.

My wish is that every woman can experience the pure ecstasy of childbirth in the way I have known it; and to know, within the deepest part of her being, that birth is not meant to be painful, dangerous, or a violation of her being ~ but that birth can be deeply transformative, empowering and orgasmic!

Birth, when celebrated in beauty and awareness, allows us to touch and glimpse the Divine. It is beautiful, inspiring, sacred, magical ~ and it is our right, as women, to birth this way. Birth isn't a competition, yet compete we do. Every woman is different, and on a unique journey. Let's celebrate women who birth from their soul and bring their babies here gently, and let us all be humble enough to learn from the wise Birthkeepers. But please, let us never, ever forget the women who, for whatever reason, didn't get to experience ecstasy in birth. Sometimes they will not want to hear our beautiful birth stories, for they are simply too painful for their wounded bodies and minds. Never doubt that by healing our own births, we're helping to heal ALL births, and to break free of cultural conditioning and messages which scream out that birth is dangerous and deadly. So, here's to my birthing systers ~ and here's to those who've yet to be initiated into the miracle we call joyous, ecstatic and beautiful birthing. I wish you well.

Veronika Sophia Robinson
Autumn, 2008. Eden Valley, Cumbria, Northern England.

The story of our ancestresses

Our ancestresses birthed alone. In fact, for most of human history, women have birthed alone. It's only in the past few centuries that birth has been attended by others, including midwives, and, more recently, men and machines. How did our ancestresses birth without medical intervention or midwives and doctors, we might wonder, when modern medicine and the dominant birth model have us believing that women need doctors if they wish to remain safe in birth?

Anthropologists who've studied cultures where women were well-fed and watered, nurtured and cared for, have found no incidence of death in childbirth for such women. Humanity has been birthing unassisted since the beginning of evolution. If birth is the dangerous, medical condition that we've been indoctrinated to believe, we simply wouldn't have survived as a species.

Some modern women are beginning to see through the dominant birth model, and are questioning many of the messages which are fed to them through antenatal care and the media. The fact is, most babies born throughout the world today, do so without being delivered into medical hands.

Women who reclaim the ancient birthing tradition of unobserved birth are finding that, contrary to popular opinion, birth is mysteriously magical, empowering and a joy.

In her study of over 500 tribal cultures, Judith Goldsmith found that the wisdom of these people manifested in a distinguishable lack of complications in childbirth. Her study found that the first people to report on tribal childbirth said "the women found it easy to give birth". One such person was Adriaen Vander Donck. He visited North America is 1641, and said the natives were rarely sick from childbirth, nor did they suffer inconvenience, or die on such occasions. This observation is common in many parts of the world. Another report, from 1884, by George Engelmann, stated that a physician who lived for eight years among the Canadian Indians saw no accidents or deaths from childbirth.

The stories continue: another doctor, who lived among the Oregon Indians, said he was never called upon to perform any serious procedure in childbirth. In Fiji, malpresentation is uncommon. The Ugandan birthing experience shows that death in childbirth is almost unknown, and rarely is there any difficulty. The Araicanians, of Argentina, state that stillbirths are a rare event, and premature birth, too, is rare.

We've been led to believe that midwifery is the oldest profession, but this is a romanticised notion, and not a fact. It is perpetuated by practitioners of midwifery and childbirth. When assisted and observed births did start becoming common place in our history, the attendant was not a specialist in birth, but most usually the mother of the woman in labour.

It appears, according to anthropologist Judith Goldsmith, that the early European writers assumed such attendants were midwives. These assumptions were based on their own backgrounds. So, if women around the world were not assisted by midwives, or other specialists in childbirth, then history shows us that birth usually does not require medical help, except in very rare cases. Throughout the 1700s and 1800s, many accounts came in from explorers showing that indigenous peoples found childbirth to be a simple event ~ calm, uncomplicated and allowed to happen in its own time. Even at that time in our history, women were bearing children without pain and suffering. The midwives of early colonised America rarely saw difficulties in birth. One in particular, who kept a diary of the births she attended between 1778 and 1812, showed only one death in childbirth ~ and that was after nine years of practice. Midwife Martha Moore said that childbirth was routinely successful.

Sleeping during birth

Women from the Tlinget of Alaska have even been known to sleep while giving birth. Indeed, there is much anthropological evidence gathered by Judith Goldsmith to indicate that traditional births were not riddled with pain as is common in Western births.

Morning sickness

Morning sickness is synonymous with pregnancy, and yet if we look to the world's oldest cultures we see that it appeared very infrequently. Much of this can be tied to the fact that their diets were simple, and their environment was clean. Morning sickness usually occurs because we no longer have the avenue of menstruation to release the build up of toxins in the body. The nausea felt is often due to such toxins being released into the blood, or of the woman not being fully accepting of the pregnancy (even if consciously planned).

Exercise

Our tribal sisters remained active throughout the length of their pregnancy, and continued to contribute to communal life. Their day to day jobs ensured all muscles were exercised in an optimal way for giving birth. They certainly didn't sit around unnecessarily or sit in front of a computer each day from 9 till 5.

Role of midwife

Although midwifery evolved from the role of birth supporter, most cultures believed that any woman who had been through childbirth herself was capable of acting as a midwife. Eventually, though, in most cultures, there would always be some women who stood out as being better skilled at supporting a birthing woman.

Often, too, it would be older women who were better able to predict challenges in childbirth. Alongside such awareness, was the implementation of herbal knowledge, which proved to be very beneficial for a birthing mother. Each tribe had its own locally grown herbs from which to draw their medicine remedy kit.

Complications

For tribal women, the rarity of a complication in childbirth can be put down to the fact they were in very good physical condition, both through moderate daily exercise, and a carefully chosen, bland, vegetarian diet. It's intriguing that so many of the common complications which make life difficult for modern women, such as high blood pressure, oedema, toxaemia, eclampsia, high blood sugar levels, and viruses such as genital herpes, were almost unknown to our tribal sisters.

Always worth bearing in mind is that although problems can happen in reproduction, the complications of childbirth are minimal if we compare them to those which result from medically-managed and manipulated births.

Our ancestresses were patient. We can learn from them, and remember that patience is the greatest midwife.

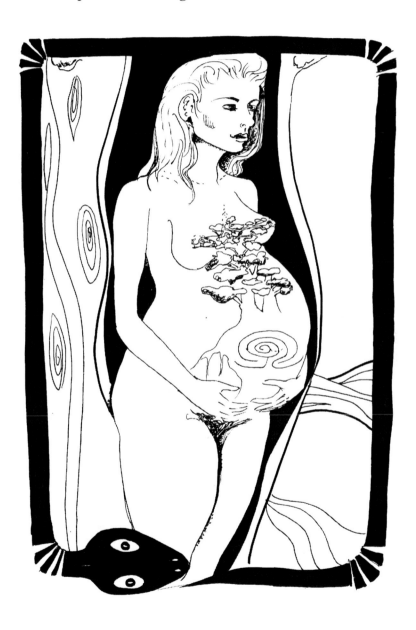

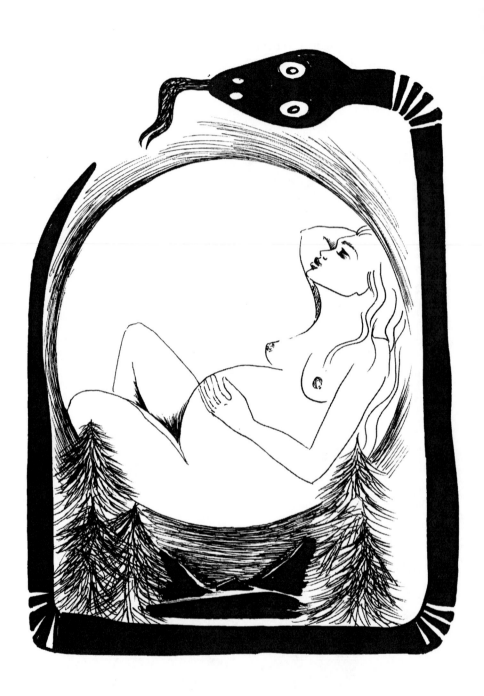

From isolation to observation

Since the 17th century, it has become commonplace for a male doctor to enter the birth room. By moving away from unobserved birth, then to birth occurring in the women's domain, and then to medicalise birth, we've seen a natural event become dangerous and feared.

Let me be clear from the outset of this chapter: this book is not anti-midwife. Midwife, in many languages, means mother. And this is what a midwife originally was ~ a mother, ideally our own, who attended us in childbirth. This, of course, is recent in human history. The purpose of this mother ~ midwife ~ was not to deliver the baby, but to act as a protector of the birth space. However, modern day professional midwifery is, for the most part, not protecting the birth space, but bringing interventions, or at the very least, the intention of intervention. And this is a very important point.

Many midwives, or medwives, as they're becoming increasingly known, are bringing danger with them because of their belief system that women need them in order to be able to birth the baby. It is this erroneous belief that has brought dissatisfaction to many birthing women, and is, ironically, leading the way for more women to give birth unobserved. If more midwives reclaimed the role of protectress, and sat on their hands during birthing, then they might be more readily welcomed into the birthing home. The ideal midwife is invisible ~ she doesn't touch, or observe with her eyes. She listens with her intuition, ears and heart, preferably in an adjacent room.

While midwives are taught about our physiological make-up, and how the body 'works' in birth, they are, in almost all cases, not skilled or trained in any way to understand how you, as a unique woman, function. They don't know your deepest needs, desires, fears or hopes. Sometimes we don't even consciously know them ourselves, until we go into birthing.

A midwife does not know which position you will feel most comfortable in; and she doesn't know what you want to see, hear, smell or feel in birth. Even with the most consciously prepared birth plan in the world, until the moment of birthing begins, no woman can truly know what she'll desire in birth or how those needs and desires might change during the course of labour.

When midwives, like doctors, feel that they are necessary for birth, we find their belief system painting the picture of the birth. In my role as editor of The Mother magazine, one of the main things I make women aware of is that if they are choosing a caregiver, it must be someone who believes birth is good, sacred and natural. As soon as you hire or invite someone in who believes it to be dangerous, or whose case history shows emergency referrals, please find someone else. Always ask them about their birthing history. How did she birth her children? What is the transfer rate among her clients? How many have ended up in hospital? How many have ended up with forceps, ventouse, caesarean? These statistics will tell you everything you need to know about your potential caregiver's beliefs about birth, and the 'baggage' she carries with her from birth to birth. Her fears and doubts will be felt within every birth scene she participates in.

Birth is not dangerous to women who are healthy, nurtured and believe birth to be safe.

This book is about encouraging you to become your own midwife, even if you choose to have one present. Know that you have within you the ability to give birth. For thousands of generations, women have done this! You carry in your cells the sacred understanding and knowing that you are the expert of your ability to give birth.

Why do women choose unobserved birth?

Childbirth:
if you want the job done right,
do it yourself!
Laura Kaplan Shanley, author, Unassisted Childbirth

Probably the first question on most people's minds when they come across the idea of unobserved and autonomous childbirth, is why would a woman choose to do this? The question itself provides the answer, as it is a guide to the mindset of most people in Western culture. We've been indoctrinated with media images of birth being the worst sort of pain imaginable. Since tv shows were first made, women have been pictured flat on their backs, sometimes strapped down, legs in stirrups and held up in the air. These images usually include women screaming in pain. Not a pretty sight by any stretch of the imagination, and the worst possible position for a woman to give birth.

If these are the images which teach us, our daughters and sisters about birth, then it would make sense to have every pain-relieving drug on the menu. It takes a deeper understanding of the mysteries of childbirth to find that birth isn't meant to be painful, frightening and unbearable.

I love the saying that "One of the greatest secrets about childbirth is not that it is painful beyond measure, but that women are powerful beyond measure".

I believe it is the fear of a woman's birthing power that has led to the widespread use of drugs and tools to control and tame this primordial strength.

Women are kept in a state of fear by having the 'birth is painful' myth perpetuated over and over again. We do this in literature, all forms of media, and, worst of all, from woman to woman, and mother to daughter. It's unusual for a pregnant woman to get to birth without having been assaulted by a battery of violent birth stories. Most modern births can only be described in that way: violent.

Violence to mother and baby is perpetrated in many, many ways.
For example:

[] Scans
[] Dopplers
[] Feeling the cervix
[] A professional touching baby's head when she is crowning
[] Forceps
[] Ventouse
[] Slashing the vagina with scissors
[] Caesareans
[] Being taken away from mother at birth for routine
   tests and procedures
[] Eye drops, vitamin K, washing and swaddling
[] Bright lights, such as fluorescent tubes
[] Clanging metal containers
[] Loud voices, irrelevant chatter, non-observance of
   the birth space as sacred

Being supported by other women, either relatives or midwives, is a very recent 'intervention'. Having birth managed by doctors and obstetricians has only been happening for half a blink of the eye in human history. The attendance of a birth care professional is still not seen in mainstream circles as an intervention. But it is, most surely, as are a pair of forceps, a Doppler, urine test, scan or scalpel. Attendants intervene by the intrusive act of observation.

People often evangelise doctors and say they 'saved' their baby. I will always disagree with that. If a baby survives birth (or any other life/death event) the doctor or midwife is a catalyst, not a life saver. It is incredibly misguided to think that a human being has the ability to keep a body and soul connected. It's simply not possible. This world we see is but a mere shadow of an unseen, real world. None of us has control over when the Light goes out, or indeed, when it begins. When we can understand, at the deepest level, that birth and death are aspects of the same thing, then we'll have unlocked one of life's deepest mysteries, and we'll let go of birth management. Society will inevitably change (for the better) as a result. I believe that most freebirth women have made the birth/death connection.

Natural birth is a place which invites nurturing and love ~ words, and a practice, not part of the obstetrical thesaurus. Birth 'care', as conducted by obstetricians, is aggressive by the very nature of it being controlling and invasive. To reclaim birth as the sacred experience gifted to us by the Goddess, we need to let go of this obsession with judging a birthing woman by her age, the size of her pelvis, previous birth history, urine samples, blood sugar levels, and so on. These are irrelevant to how she'll give birth. What we really need to look at is how she was born. How did her mother bring her into the world? Our own birth has a huge impact on how we approach bringing children into the world ~ consciously or otherwise. We will either repeat or heal our own birth when we re-birth with our children.

The reason our culture advocates medically-supervised birth is because it wants women controlled; for, without doubt, there is nothing more primal (or beautiful) than an empowered birthing woman. Sadly, most medics are in denial about our mammalian needs in birth, and therefore, can't see that their interventions, or the threat of them, are what cause birth to be dangerous.

How is it that women usually manage to conceive without interference ~ though this is changing dramatically in these modern, soul-less times ~ but can't give birth without 'help'? Both conception and birth are sacred and otherworldly miracles made manifest in the physical. Perhaps if more people start witnessing conception as a conscious, creative, selfless act of intimacy, in which they first discover themselves, we'd see it mirrored in an easy, pain-free, spontaneous birth, also.

Women choose autonomous birth for many reasons. One is that by being in her own home, without being answerable to a midwife or doctor, she can move in a way that feels comfortable to her, and eat or drink when she wants to. She can take up different birthing positions which feel right to her. What she is doing, by giving birth alone, is listening to her inner guidance, rather than seeking approval and affirmation from an external source. This same inner guidance (the innate intelligence) is what created her baby from an egg and sperm. This guidance has grown her baby throughout gestation.

One reason for an unassisted birth is for the moments after, when it is naturally time for the mother to hold her baby, and breastfeed. By not being observed, she will birth as easily as possible, and bond with her baby in the way Nature intended.

One of the most damaging things which happens in the moments after a medically-supervised birth is the removal of the baby from the mother for routine tests.

In these precious moments, when the baby should be in his mother's arms having skin to skin contact and access to the breast, the child is learning that the world is not a safe place. Millions of years of human evolution have etched within babe's cells that he should be breastfeeding. And mother, too, is expecting this, whether she is aware of it or not.

By hindering the commencement of suckling in the newborn, we subdue the old brain. Our newborn baby is forced to slip into using the neo-cortex (new brain) at the very time he needs to be engaged in primitive instincts, such as taking in the smell of mother, breastfeeding, and skin to skin contact. Research shows self-destructive behaviours such as violence, suicide, drug addiction, anorexia, and the condition of autism in children, all have in common a disturbed birth. By interfering with the stimulation of oxytocin ~ the hormone of love ~ we are short-circuiting maternal love. This is being played out every day in Western hospitals (and increasingly in developing countries), and is changing the face of civilisation. We're losing the ability to love, because we were deprived of it at birth. It was stolen from us by a paranoid medical team which believed eye drops, vitamin K injections, weighing, swaddling, and taking blood pressure were more important than bonding. Biologically, nothing is more important than bonding with our mother.

Even if a woman chooses to give birth alone, the truth is, for her, that she is accompanied by the Creator ~ whatever term you use for describing All That Is. She fully feels inner guidance with her through birth, and therefore doesn't feel alone. All birthing women have access to this, but in order to hear and feel this inner power/ comforter and companion, they must close off the outside world.

Home sweet homebirth

Our home is a place of nurturing. The familiar smells, sounds and objects create a space of love. Our feeling nature, the love we've shared in our home, emanate from the walls and furnishings. Our heart plays here. It is where we feel safe. It is the ideal place to give birth, in freedom. Women can feel empowered and share intimate moments with their life partner here, without intrusive procedures being carried on, or around, them. Anyone who works with mammals will tell you that they don't birth as easily, or breastfeed as successfully, when they are observed. It's the same for human mammals.

It would be far too easy and convenient to lump freebirthing women into a single category of hippy Earth mums, and to not give credit to their birth awareness. Freebirthers are more informed and aware of the birthing process than any other birthing group. For many of them, their research, awareness and studies began well before conception. I believe what they tend to have in common is the awareness of the Divine, as Jeannine Parvati Baker described: a new breed of human called Homo Divinitus.

In the past few decades, thousands of Western mothers have chosen freebirth. Changing ideas about birth, the idea of taking full responsibility for it, and a deeper understanding of mind, body and soul, health and well-being, are contributing to this deep sea-change in how we view birthing.

In choosing to take responsibility, a freebirthing woman will understand and recognise possible complications and how to deal with them. She will be knowledgeable about first aid, self-care, and medical back-up, should it be necessary. Contrary to popular opinion, she is not ignorant or putting her baby at unnecessary risk.

Freebirthers rarely have unresolved complications when compared to 'observed' birthing women.

Why doesn't anyone tell a mother who opts for scans, drugs, forceps, ventouse or a caesarean, being observed (our mammalian brain registers everything!), that she is potentially putting herself and her baby in 'grave' danger? Why isn't she warned that the risks greatly outweigh the benefits? Why are these women not questioned about their birthing choices?

I believe it is for two very simple reasons:

1.) Women birthing under the medical model are in the majority, and it is the cultural norm to give all responsibility to the medical profession. Those women are, therefore, completely exempt from taking any responsibility for the outcome: good, bad or deeply traumatic.

2.) There's no money for birth professionals when a woman gives birth unassisted. The more intervention in a birth, the more money the doctor or obstetrician makes. There is absolutely no incentive for doctors, obstetricians and medwives to understand natural, unobserved birth.

We've become so far removed from our biological design that we can't even recognise Nature's perfection. We need to stop looking for what's wrong, and look for what's right.

Studies into the common, significant factors shared by autistic children are sobering. Although there are more than 20 factors, these children often have at least four or five in common, including:
[] Deep forceps delivery
[] Separation of mother and child at birth (this always happens after birth problems)
[] Being hospitalised in early life
[] Being exposed to too many strange faces in the early years

Every invention that a mother accepts as normal will separate her from her child, such as:
[] A pregnancy test (rather than listening to her body tell her that she's pregnant)
[] Scans to tell her that baby is growing and is ok (rather than intuition)
[] Antenatal tests (the usual barrage: urine, blood, heart)
[] Drugs to 'mask' her fear
[] Fake milk for babe (this topic is so huge and fundamentally explosive to humans, personally and collectively, and humanity's future, that it takes a book to discuss it ~ see The Drinks Are On Me)
[] Cots, cribs, prams, day-care, early institutional learning

These put a physical, emotional and spiritual distance between mother and child. The trouble is that this numbing-out becomes the norm, and our detachment is not questioned. Rather, those with a strong mothering instinct are made to look abnormal, clingy, smothering.

If women are honest, there's nothing encouraging or supportive about hearing horrific birth stories. So why do we keep perpetuating them? And why does the media keep showing women flat on their backs in birth? It's the worst possible position! If you choose the medical system, and eat rubbish, drink alcohol, smoke, don't rest adequately, work throughout your pregnancy, don't exercise, stay in a negative relationship, etc., you're ok. The system will take care of you and pick up the pieces. It is rarely questioned.

Only a small number of complications occur in birth that couldn't have been predicted in pregnancy. And for these, it is rare that an obstetrician would be needed.

It is statistically safer for mother and baby to birth at home than in a hospital. I find it very interesting that most women who choose to birth unassisted actually know more about the act of childbirth than the average medical student does. Midwives and doctors don't grow babies for people. They are not omnipotent. Sometimes a complication can be detected and dealt with before it becomes a problem, and sometimes it can't, regardless of technology. Ultimately, God/dess (All That Is) has the final say.

Mammalian Birth

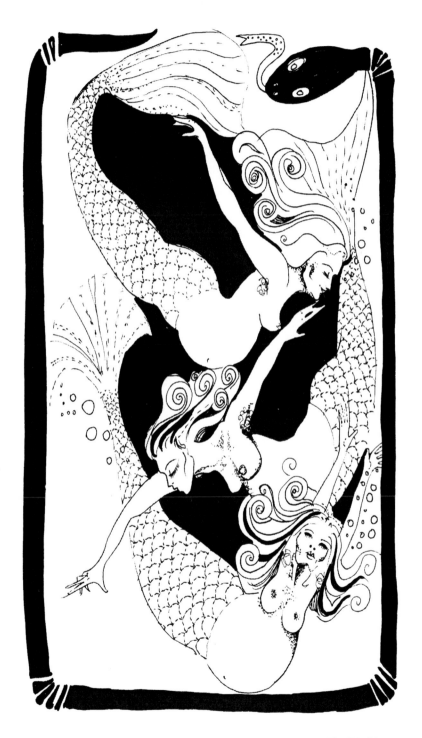

From my experience of talking to women who are preparing for an autonomous childbirth, I would say that all of them have done so knowing that they had to take 100% responsibility for their actions. They've taken great care with their health and well-being, usually doing so from before conception. These women nurture mind, body and soul. For them it's a priority to surround themselves with positive influences and uplifting birth stories. Many of them understand the mind/body connection and how the thoughts we constantly think, or the beliefs we hold, shape our reality.

When it comes to defining joyous freebirth, it's important to understand the role of power. I believe the difference between an interfered-with birth, and a joyous, hands-off birth, is fear. Fear can come from a deep primal urge in the old brain, or from our centre of logic (the neo-cortex or new brain) ~ a place where we try to make sense of the unexplainable. Our ego freaks out when it can't control the information. Taming our powerful ego empowers us.

In the dominant cultural model of birth, the leading actor is The Obstetric Observer, who 'delivers' our baby. In the sub-culture of joyous, autonomous birth, the leading role is played by The Birthkeeper. Indeed, there is no place for The Obstetric Observer in this culture.

Never will you find such different characters. In fact, they are so diametrically opposed, that you would never find them both in the same room ~ much less on the same birthing stage. The only connection might be if, through the performance of The Obstetric Observer, a woman becomes transformed, at a later time, into a Birthkeeper. Their props, their scripts, their guiding drives are polar opposites.

The Obstetric Observer comes into being through domination. S/he conquers the other characters by taking charge of the stage and wielding tools which say "I'm in charge". He is defined by his use of three specific tools. They are light, language and observation. Whether he is conscious of this or not is irrelevant, because as soon as they are introduced into the delivery room, his status is confirmed.

Light is the enemy of every birthing woman. It stimulates her 'new brain', and changes the course of labour. Her mammalian instincts wish to seek out the dark, but The Obstetric Observer shines a laser beam on her, freezing her in time like a startled rabbit in headlights.

He controls her by his use of language, which activates her neo-cortex (new brain).

While this is engaged and stimulated, she is incapable of slipping into her mammalian brain ~ the very place she needs to be in order to birth instinctively. The Obstetric Observer stands guard over the woman whose baby he's delivering. If he can't be there, he sends others to guard her, lest she escape and prove she doesn't need him. Their eyes ensure that she can't escape. She is watched. Her every movement observed. She is held in place by their paranoia. Privacy is the number one need of every birthing woman. The Obstetric Observer denies this, keeping a woman prisoner in her new brain so she can't meet her baby without his help.

Light, language and observation ~ the three deadly enemies of joyous, freebirth. And what of The Birthkeeper? What would she make of these tools? She's a wise woman, who, like the three wise monkeys, has her own mantra:

See no light
Hear no talk
Allow no eyes

The Birthkeeper is a woman who honours the ancient tradition of birthing. She creates a birthing nest under dimmed light, if not complete darkness. The external language of choice is non-vaginal touch, or music, chanting, or gentle singing, as she slips into her birthing zone. If she chooses to have her lover, or anyone else with her, she lets them know beforehand that eye contact is another form of power, of control. The support she seeks is of skin contact, and being held from behind.

Beware of any man or midwife who demands or encourages you to look into their eyes while you're birthing. Contrary to our culture's childbirth classes, these birth attendants are stealing your inner power. Remember, our eyes are the mirror of our soul. When we're birthing, our soul needs to rise 'upwards' and greet the new soul who is coming Earthside. We should not be distracted by someone else's needs: that is, their need to feel like they're controlling how you give birth, or their need to feel important in the unfolding of events. This may be unconsciously driven, or be ego-based.

The Birthkeeper is clear to her supporter that all the power she needs for birthing is within her, and that coaching, of any description, defies what is innate to her. The instinct to give birth is always heard by those with ears to hear. Sadly, joyous birth is inaudible to The Obstetric Observer.

It has been said that 'when the power of love overcomes the love of power, there shall be peace'. It has also been said that 'peace on Earth begins with birth'. True power and true peace are internal and can never be found outside ourselves. The Birthkeeper is a woman whose power is always internal. Instinct is beyond anyone's control. It can't be bought, begged, borrowed or stolen. Perhaps that's why it terrifies the medical world so much. The Obstetric Observer requires tools, gimmicks and fear to build his arsenal of power ~ something which is always external, and therefore, transient.

The power of love, which is alive in The Birthkeeper, can teach us more about birth than any medical text book. Love and fear can't co-exist. They are opposites.

We've been inculturated with the idea that birth is painful, dangerous and deadly. I agree. It is painful, dangerous and deadly IF, and only if, we allow The Obstetric Observer
into our birthing space: if we give away our crucial mammalian need for privacy.

In media interviews I like to use the 'making love' analogy to try and explain the requirements for a birthing woman. I do so in the hope people might be able to relate to their own experiences of intimacy. This, of course, can only make some sense to people for whom love and sex have not become desensitised in any way by pornographic viewing and perpetration, lust, drugs and alcohol.

When we make love, we do so best in the dark or semi-dark, in an atmosphere conducive to our hormones working well. We need comforting smells and touch, whispered voices. In essence, we need to be wooed. If you were making love to your partner and they suddenly stopped to turn on the tv for cricket results, or raced out of the room to stop the toast burning, or just when you were ready to orgasm, your mum phone ~ well, it would disrupt the whole experience. The flow would be interrupted. The same hormones are used in birth and breastfeeding. We're simply not designed to have strangers watching us when we give birth, any more than we're designed to have our blood pressure or heart checked, fingers checking our cervix, etc. It's unnatural. It's wrong!

Most hospital births, by their very nature, involve fluorescent lighting, metal dishes being banged around, staff talking to each other, the bloody clock on the wall, machines beeping, invasive vaginal checks, etc. What sort of an environment is that in which to welcome a sacred being Earthside, or to help a mother submit to the mood, beauty and sanctity of birth? It reeks of something rather barbaric. Studies show that if birth is violent, then violence is much more likely to be part of life later on. Muck around with birth and you're asking for trouble. Every intervention is an intervention on the pathway to more intervention. Accept it at your own risk.

Don't worry though, because no-one will call you irresponsible, even if you've never given it any thought or your informed consent. No-one will call you irresponsible when your baby is handled like a lump of meat, rather than the exquisitely sensitive being she is.

There are only three words a birthing woman needs to remember if she wishes to keep her experience safe and sacred: darkness, privacy, silence.

Could it really be so simple? Yes. Absolutely, completely, positively, YES.

Should everyone have an unassisted childbirth? No, I don't believe so. We've been so indoctrinated with medical beliefs and false media impressions of birth, that some women simply wouldn't be able to turn their thinking around in order to create that sort of birth. It may take more than a few generations to remind us that birth can be easy, natural and pain free. However, if women in the dominant medical model were afforded more privacy, darkness and silence ~ as well as only being shown positive birth images and stories ~ we would see difficulties in childbirth fall away rapidly. Women who choose to have assistants at birth can learn a lot from The Birthkeepers. That lesson is very much about self-belief and not underestimating your own abilities. Looking within, listening within, rather than outside ourselves, is the key to a flowing birth. It is this moving within, rediscovering our intuition, that shows us our power.

Damsel in distress
The worlds between pleasure and pain

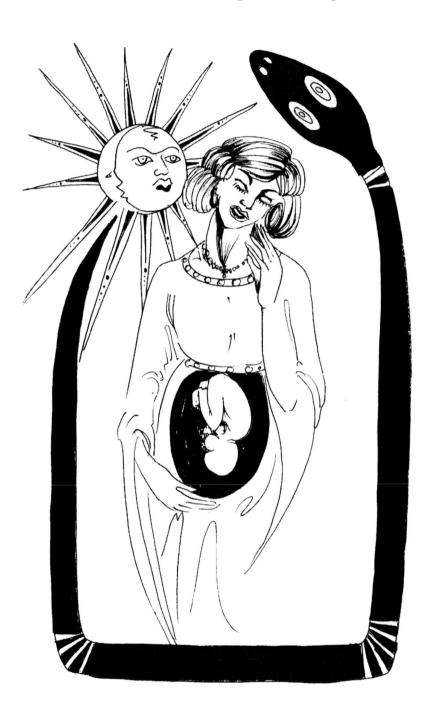

At The Mother magazine, our ethos regarding birth is that we don't wish to perpetuate the belief that birth is 'dangerous or painful', but rather, that birth can be beautiful, ecstatic and indeed, orgasmic, just as Nature intended.

A lot of women have difficulty with this statement, either because that hasn't been their experience, and, so far, they've not had the opportunity to expand their frame of reference, or because they've been so indoctrinated by fear or belief systems, that they would feel naked without the badge of honour that says "I gave birth, and it hurt like hell!" or "The doctor saved my baby's life". Sadly, many women feel that birth isn't real, or that they haven't gone through some sort of rite of passage, if birth is pleasurable and ecstatic. We simply don't need to go through tragedy, pain or difficult times in order to grow: to be more of who we are.

I don't buy the often touted biblical assertion (another of culture's invisible messages) that childbirth pain is the legacy of sin, any more than I believe our culture's script of 'birth is dangerous and painful'.

It's not just birthing women who perpetuate the pain and danger of childbirth, midwives do so, too. Every time we say 'birth is painful' or 'dangerous', we are poisoning the minds of mothers, sisters and daughters the world over. Yes, birth can be intense, but please, let's use the right language. If we want to look at why women think birth is painful, then we have to be honest about what they've experienced, and put it into perspective.

Have you ever witnessed an animal stuck in a man-made metal trap? Have you heard it screaming or howling in pain? When a woman is chained to an IV drip; is strapped like a mentally-challenged patient to a metal table; has her legs hoisted up in stirrups like an animal in a slaughterhouse; when her baby is pulled out with a barbaric metal tool or forcefully by suction; when her sensitive and tender vagina is slashed by razor-sharp scissors because her instinctively-confused body is no longer in a position to birth as Nature intended, then yes, you will hear screams of pain. I would never pretend otherwise, but let's be clear and honest, this isn't birth as Nature intended for humans. This is torture, birth rape, cruelty. This is medically (mis)managed delivery of a baby. And let's not forget, babies are extremely sensitive. It is a complete denial and ignorance of what a birthing mammal and her young need. Birth, as Nature intended, does not cause pain, and it certainly does not lead to a woman sounding like a brutally-tortured animal.

How can we be so culturally dumb and numb to this? That we suffer pain is a direct reflection of our fear of birth and of our body ~ either our own fears, or an energetic taking-on of ancestral wounds from recent times. We carry cellular memories from when matriarchal societies were overruled and nine million witches (aka wise women!) were burned for knowing about women's power (birth, menstruation, herbs, dreams, etc.). That's a rather heavy burden for females to carry, but it doesn't mean we need to create invasive, violent or disrespectful births. We can change the pattern. And we need to, for the sake of humanity. Women, such as The Birthkeepers, are taking this into their hands. All praise to them, because each woman who brings a baby into this world gently, peacefully and magically, is helping to change the collective energy around birth. I have nothing but deep admiration for them.

If you choose to give birth in hospital, it's important to understand that labour is at least ten times more intense (painful) when a woman is given the drug Pitocin.

When a birth professional controls what a woman eats or drinks in labour, the mother-to-be may end up not getting what she needs. This lowers her tolerance for dealing with labour.

A hospital environment impedes a woman's instincts to find positions which are most comfortable for her. It will also cause the release of adrenalin (a stress hormone), which will inhibit her ability to birth naturally. It makes labour last for longer, and she is very likely, in this environment, to feel pain.

Pharmaceutical drugs are not the be all and end all in creating a painless childbirth. They do, in fact, bring hazards and side-effects to mother and baby, and should be avoided at all costs.

The first tool on any Birthkeeper's list should be the practice of visualisation. Our imagination is what creates our reality. Every thought we think creates our future. Some women prefer prayer, and others, still, prefer to affirm their birthing outcome. Placing words on cards around the home brings certain ideas or beliefs into focus, and, more importantly, into the subconscious. Helpful words include: easy, gentle, peaceful, smooth, open, loving. In either a home or hospital environment, a woman can use natural methods to ease her labour, such as a birth pool, hypnotherapy (practised during pregnancy), herbs, flower essences, acupressure, position changes, rocking, walking, belly dancing.

The most helpful way of providing natural comfort in labour is by submersion in a warm water birthing tub. The warmth of the water is comforting, and the water itself provides relief from gravity. Buoyancy can be a birthing girl's best friend. Some women have found that physical intimacy with their partner, or self-pleasuring, helps trigger the birthing hormones. It's often said that women have two sets of lips: one above and one below. For relaxed birthing, both sets of lips need to be relaxed. Kissing helps this enormously! As does singing. Try and get into the practice of singing throughout your pregnancy, and draw on this during labour. And as mentioned, affirmations, prayers, and visualisations are invaluable. But ultimately, I believe that birth is not painful or dangerous in and of itself. Generations of fear, shame, and guilt, however, make it so for many women in Western culture.

Fear equals danger,
and even if there is no danger
in the birth,
those who are feeling fear
will create anxiety
in mother and child.

There's nothing to fear...

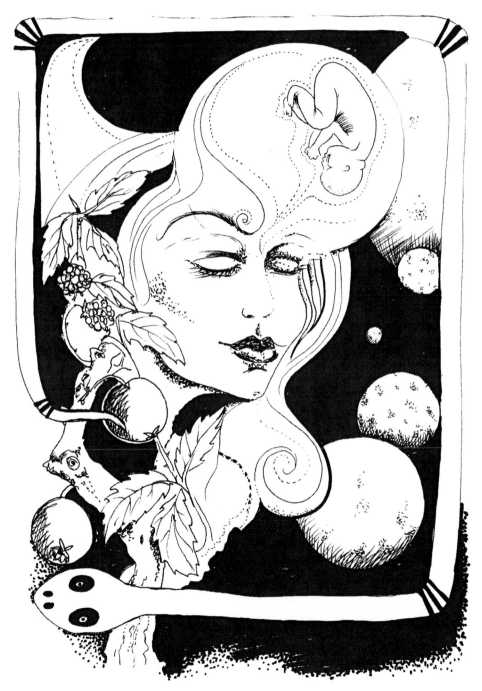

As a child, my mother often told me that "there's nothing to fear, but fear itself". I believe she borrowed the phrase from a former American president. These words have stood me in good stead throughout life, allowing me to challenge myself, and take risks when necessary.

Grantly Dick-Read, author of Childbirth without Fear, believed, as I do, that Nature created women to give birth painlessly and easily. He stated that this happens when we're unafraid.

The most deadly thing anyone can bring to the birthing room is fear. It may be invisible, but it seeps into every corner, and into the body of everyone present. Fear equals danger, and even if there is no danger in the birth, those who are feeling fear will create anxiety in mother and child. For a birthing woman, this means that her body will go into fight or flight mode. In fight mode, her body will send all the oxygen and blood to her arms and legs. This gives her the ability to run from the 'perceived' danger (doctor?), or fight it. However, she can only do this because all the bodily functions considered to be non-essential will close down. One such function is the use of our sexual organs. When the uterus is denied blood and oxygen, it causes pain. Our body is trying to protect us from what it perceives as danger e.g. doctor, midwives, lights, noise, machines, eyes…Birth isn't meant to be painful. It is meant to be ecstatic, joyous and free. Free, in particular, from fear. Dr. Crippen (possibly a pseudonym) is a British National Health Service doctor who claims that "giving birth is the most dangerous thing that most women will do during their life".

Many people say that birth is as safe as life gets! Hospitals are not, as we are encouraged to believe, the safest place to give birth. The reason so many women have died in childbirth was not because birth was dangerous, but because of the standard of living at the time. Women lived on the poverty line, were undernourished, and most certainly were overworked in pregnancy.

In England, the wealthy women were kept indoors as brown (tanned) skin was not fashionable. Corsets were popular; however, they caused major problems to the pelvis, and meant young women couldn't birth easily. A study of childbirth history is revealing. It shows that only when birth moved away from home to hospital, circa 1920s, did we see a rise in maternal mortality. Studies since then have affirmed that homebirths are safer.

It's all in the mind

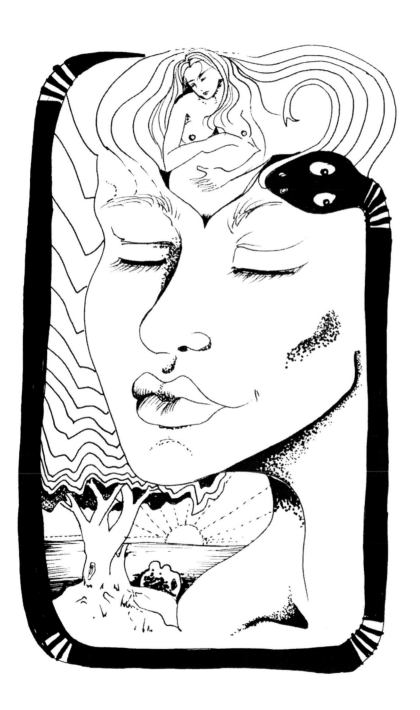

As already discussed, fear is an enemy of pleasurable birth. Grantly Dick-Read said the uterus of a frightened woman in labour is 'white' (because it is drained of blood and oxygen). Giving birth is so intimately linked to our sexuality, that if we have any issues or hang-ups in this area, they almost certainly manifest in how we view and experience birth. If we believe (at any level) that women shouldn't enjoy sex or pleasure, then we, too, will believe birth shouldn't be enjoyable.

In order to create a joyous birth we must love, nurture and respect our body. We can get an inkling into our beliefs about sex and our body by examining our menstrual cycle. Is it a time of ease, reflection and self-care, or is it a week of the month disguised by industrial strength painkillers? Do we take time out from the world to take care of our emotional, physical and spiritual needs, or do we act as if we're 'men', continuing our life as if nothing is going on?

Despite the cultural and media images of birth as dangerous and painful, we can change our beliefs around this. This is where visualisation, meditation, affirmations and journaling (to be explained later) come into their own. We can choose to believe that, instead of birth needing to be assisted by doctors and midwives, and instead of tools like forceps, ventouse, and scalpels greeting our baby, we can bring our child Earthside in a sacred atmosphere of love, trust, calm and peace.

Do you believe birth is safe?

Do you believe in your body?

During the pregnancy of my first daughter, I created a large vision board with what I believed to be true about birth, my body and my ideal birth. I included words and pictures.

I began by addressing my fears. These included: hospital; drugs; machines; forceps; baby taken away; picking up other people's fears or lack of concern; my beliefs not being respected; and not feeling safe. I wrote these out, and then put a cross through the page to let my mind know that the fears held no power over me.

I wrote what I expected:

[] our baby being born gently, peacefully, and welcomed into a
   loving, happy and safe environment
[] I take full responsibility for my birthing
[] dim lights/candlelight
[] relaxing music
[] familiar, caring support people
[] baby born under water
[] holding and feeding our baby straight after birth
[] for my husband to be equally present and conscious
   at our baby's birth
[] safe at home to be myself

I wrote a list of all the things I could do to prepare myself for birthing. I drew pictures of flowers showing my cervix fully open. Inside,
it held the belief "it is safe to open and share our beautiful baby with
the world in an easy, gentle and peaceful birthing".

Another flower, pasted to my fridge, contained one word: OPEN.
I left affirmations all around the house. They included:

[] our baby is developing perfectly
[] we can communicate with our baby at all times
[] our child is pure, sacred and holy
[] birthing is a time of pleasure
[] there is nothing to be feared
[] the movements of my uterus hug and massage my
   baby during birthing
[] my cervix knows how to open
[] our baby descends naturally
[] the baby's head fits perfectly into my pelvis

I pasted words like: ecstasy ~ a natural high; waterbirth; a natural
healing. I kept a drawing nearby of a baby in the optimal foetal position for being born. I visualised my baby being in that position.

The Dance of Love

It's often said that birth is women's work, and that there's no place for a man in the birthing room. Such blanket statements really need exploring so clarity can reveal the essence of any potential wisdom. In times past, men were protectors of the birthing space. With their back to the woman, they kept an eye, not on her, but on any predators. This was their role.

For the last 30 or 40 years, it has become commonplace for a man to be at his wife's side during birth. And even more latterly, to act as a 'birth coach', telling her when and how to breathe! Can you see how dramatically and drastically his role in birth has changed?

As with any attendant at birth, it's important that the partner/baby's father understands what it is that a woman needs to birth easily: dim lighting; near-silence (lack of language); non-observation; and a room free of fear. His role (or hers, if you're in a lesbian partnership) is best served by holding you gently from behind (if, and only if, you desire it).

Just as a picture can paint a thousand words, so too, can touch. His gentle presence is all that you need. He doesn't need to do anything. Basics, such as towels, warm water, etc., should be attended to before birthing commences.

A woman does not need busyness around her, and she certainly doesn't need to be told how to breathe or push. Birth is instinctive, and if left alone, a woman will automatically do these things.

Birth is a reflection of the relationship we have with our partner. When inviting (or expecting) our partner/lover/husband/the baby's father to our birth, we need to make time for honesty, to see if there are underlying issues which need resolving. Anything that causes tension, e.g. money, either between you, or for you both, should be addressed before birth. If birth is going to be your mirror, what does your life need to be showing? How can you gently create a relationship of love, harmony, trust and respect?

A conscious birth is a natural consequence of a conscious conception. The key word is conscious ~ and it is up to you to keep this awareness with you throughout pregnancy. When we treat our partner as if they're a king or queen, caring for them, being mindful of their needs and desires, as well as our own, a dance develops ~ it's one of beauty, harmony and love.

I recommend Breathwork (see references) for all couples before birth, to help clear birth issues. If your partner is going to attend birth, it's just as important that they clear all beliefs about birth.

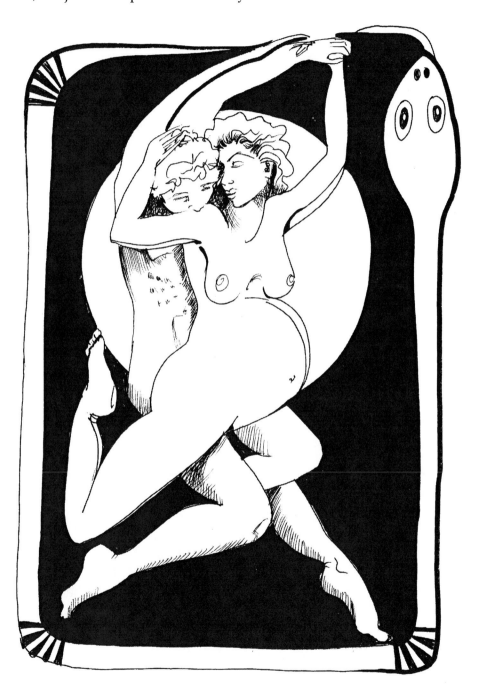

Peaceful Pregnancy

Pregnancy is Nature's sabbatical ~ a time to draw inwards, and attend to spiritual needs. You don't need to ask for permission to nurture your deepest physical, emotional, spiritual and intellectual needs. In an ideal world, your family and friends would gather around to tend to you, not because you're in any way infirm, but to affirm your body is a vessel which transports a soul Earthside into a physical body.

Pregnancy should be synonymous with a simple life. By this, I mean, attending to basic impulses. There are creative tools with which to enjoy your pregnancy journey. These include:

Journaling

Each pregnancy is a unique experience. You might like to use your journal to draw your feelings and record body changes, or you might prefer to use it as a space to write affirmations. My husband and I kept journals which were letters to our unborn children. They are now in our daughters' possession, and it is something they both treasure. Another form of journaling which I've found very beneficial is the daily practice of Morning Pages. This idea comes from Julia Cameron's book, The Artist's Way. You don't need to be a writer to do this. Simply start each day writing three foolscap (A4) pages, non-stop. Don't think, just write about whatever comes to mind. It's not about being a wordsmith, or fine-tuning every sentence that lands on the page, but letting all your thoughts, fears, feelings, joys, frustrations, anticipations, etc., get oxygen. By doing so, you're freeing up enormous reserves of energy which might well have been blocking or trapping intuitive messages. The important thing about Morning Pages is that you don't re-read them. Just put them away, and write again the next day on a fresh page. Ask yourself questions. How do I feel about being pregnant? How do I feel about birth? Do I feel supported, loved, nourished, honoured? What can I do to have my needs met? Who do I love to have around me? What inspires me? What images am I feeding my baby? Do I choose only to watch, witness and hear beautiful images and thoughts? If not, why? Am I eating in a way that fully supports me and my baby? Explore your answers. Let them take you on a journey. Don't fight what arrives on the page, but welcome it like a long lost guest. Feed your guest! Ask, 'what do I need?'

It's also worth writing with your non-dominant hand, in order to access your inner child. She might just have a thing or two to tell you.

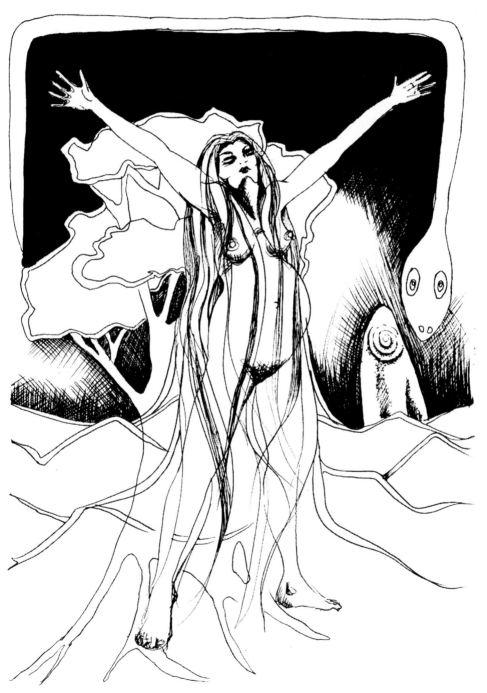

Vision board

Use positive words and colourful pictures to create a visual poster of your hopes, expectations and beliefs about pregnancy and birth. It's helpful to include words like relaxing, loved, happy, nourished. Images are so powerful, and find their way deep into our subconscious; so create a vision board that's a joy to look at ~ a visual feast! Use as much colour as you can. Some people feel a bit self-conscious about having a vision board where others can see it, so why not make a scrap book version? This way, you can look at your vision book every morning upon rising, and just before sleeping at night; and, of course, any time you wish during the day.

Yoga

Even if you've never done physical (hatha) yoga in your life, a weekly antenatal class will help to prepare you for birth. Once you become familiar with some basic moves suitable for the various stages of pregnancy, you can incorporate them into your day. They're particularly good to do just before lunch time, as an oasis of relaxation in your day.

There are many types of physical yoga, so ensure you choose a suitable class specific to pregnancy.

Aquanatal classes

Don't wait until you're waddling around before enjoying aquanatal classes. This is a fabulously refreshing and energising way to exercise during pregnancy. It uses all your muscles, without causing strain. Most towns and cities offer classes. If you have the choice, opt for a salt water pool rather than a chlorine-based one.

Walking

There's no budget which can't afford walking, and if you've got use of your legs, then this is the number one exercise for every pregnant woman. There are no restrictions. Make sure you do it regularly for maximum benefit. If at all possible, avoid doing so near heavy traffic and other stressful or polluted areas. This is meant to be a time of relaxation and enjoyment. You could purchase a step counter (very inexpensive) to have an idea of your daily walking distance. You should aim for a minimum of 5,000 steps a day. Look for glorious places in Nature to walk, such as beaches, woodlands, riversides and meadows.

Pilates

Pilates is suitable for everyone, including people who have weak abdominals, poor posture and are recovering from back problems. It gives increased flexibility, and the more often you engage in these well-designed stretching and strengthening exercises, the stronger you'll become. There are special exercises for pregnancy, and it's well worth incorporating a Pilates routine into your daily life before, during and after pregnancy. It will also pay dividends later on. Your pelvic floor muscles will thank you.

Dreams

For me, dreams are like an elixir ~ they can be magical, mysterious, revealing and full of deep insights. The more I observe them, or interact in lucid dreams, the more I learn about myself and others. Many women find that dreams give them answers to concerns and questions they may have about their baby, the birth or birthing environment. Some women also receive messages in their dreams about the position their baby will be born in, such as breech. It's always worth keeping a dream diary, and writing down as much detail as you can remember. I feel this is even more so in pregnancy, when we're more connected to the spirit world. Even if the dreams aren't prophetic, they can certainly help us to acknowledge, and let go of, our fears. Laura Shanley, author of Unassisted Childbirth, dreamt about giving birth on her hands and knees. Interestingly, while she was giving birth she realised her baby was breech. Some time later, she read that French Obstetrician, Michel Odent, recommends this as the best position for birthing a breech baby.

Conscious relaxation and mindful awareness

Many Westerners believe meditation is hard (even if they haven't even tried it!). In fact, it is very simple. It normally involves, in a relaxed manner, focusing our attention on one thing ~ such as a word (mantra), an object (for example, a flower), or the breathing ~ following the progress of the breath in and out of the body. Thoughts and tension tend to fall away. The more we practise, the easier it becomes. The calmness, peace and love which comes from being in such a space is actually how humans were designed to feel. Why would we want to fight this? Ours is a world buzzing with electromagnetic radiation from cordless phones, wi-fi, microwave ovens, mobile phones, satnav, etc. We live in an unnatural 'field'.

This was never Nature's intention for us. Although it can be fun to live the 24/7 life, it takes its toll, and stress soon eats away at our health and vitality.

Conscious relaxation is a universally available tool which clears the mind. Rather than thinking of meditation as a chore or something only for the spiritually committed, try it for a week, and see how this personal dedication to yourself changes your life.

In the end, the more humans who choose conscious relaxation and mindful awareness, the more enriched all of humanity will be, because the vibrations are so positive, and radiate to all humans.

"Beautiful birth stories only, please.
My baby is listening."

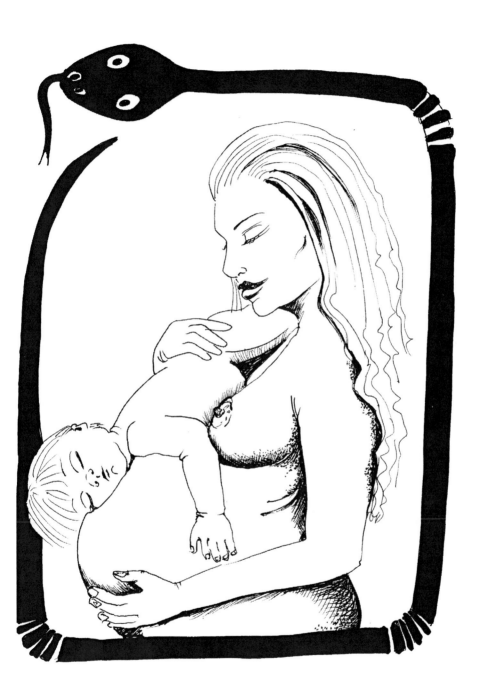

Visualisation

Along with meditation, allowing ourselves to picture, in our mind's eye, a healthy, enjoyable pregnancy and easy birthing and post-partum, is a personal and powerful antenatal ritual. You can visualise whenever you remember to, or pick aside a few minutes every day to go through your 'inner film' of easy birthing. The more you view them, the more powerful the images become, until they seep down into the subconscious and replace fears, worries and out-dated beliefs.

A birth altar provides a focal point in your home or garden. You can do this by placing symbolic images of birth and fertility ~ such as fruit, eggs, spirals, the Moon, pregnant or birthing women, perhaps modelled in clay ~ in a dedicated space.

Bellydancing

According to Egyptian history, the Pharaonic queens had birth chambers called mamisi. It was here that they would dance their way through labour, in honour of Isis, the Great Mother. Bellydancing shows us the beauty of pregnancy and birth. The movements are symbols of fertility ~ hip rocking, hip eight, hip circle. Some women use other names, like full Moon and cradle Moon.

By bellydancing, a pregnant woman can find a way to love and accept her changing shape. Her pelvic muscles are strengthened before birth, as well as her legs. It's ideal practice for birthing upright. All the movements help to release strains and stresses. Some of the chest movements are soothing for women who experience heartburn.

The baby is massaged by some of the movements, such as continuous hip circles. The dancing stimulates the uterus, which is great for bringing oxygen to the baby and your body, as well as keeping you free of fear. Bellydancing benefits all women, not just professional dancers.

I believe one of the greatest gifts of bellydancing is that it helps us to reclaim our sacred, feminine sensuality.

Singing

French obstetrician, Michel Odent, regularly led singing classes when he worked in France. This is a great idea for an antenatal group. If you haven't got a group nearby, start one.

If, like me, you're too shy to sing in front of anyone besides the local toads, then sing on your own, sing in the shower, garden, kitchen; sing fully, vibrantly, and with all your soul. Others may not like your singing, you may not even think it's that great ~ but your baby will love it!

Living simply ~ that is, having plenty of pure water, clean air, organic foods, freshly grown herbs, sleep, rest, love, laughter, time in Nature, loving touch, bellydancing, singing ~ means creating a nurturing environment in which to bathe yourself and the baby you're growing inside.

We're highly sensitive to environmental factors, and should endeavour to create a place and space of beauty in and around us. It's so much easier to care for ourselves and our unborn baby if we bring consciousness (mindful awareness) to pregnancy and birthing. It may feel indulgent to nurture our sensory self, but actually, it's a necessity. Create love, passion and sensuality as a daily feast. Everything we feed our self ~ physically, emotionally, mentally and spiritually ~ we also feed to our baby.

Pregnancy self-care is a precursor to self-care in labour and birth. In the safety and sanctity of our home we can create a love nest. We can enjoy candlelit baths, fill our space with cushions, soothing music, cups of hot chamomile or red raspberry leaf tea, and receive lavender oil massages. When the pregnant mother is nurtured, her baby is nurtured. Everything the mother feels will be transmitted to babe. Every mother should ask herself, "Is my womb a terror-filled prison for my baby ~ due to my anxiety and fears, or is it a five-star sanctuary?" Regardless of our life circumstances, we can choose to give our baby luxurious accommodation for the first nine months.

When pregnancy doesn't feel so peaceful, we need to question the areas in our life where self-care is being neglected. Are we getting enough nutrients, exercise, sleep, relaxation, love, friendship, companionship, solitude? One of the most common ailments in pregnancy is nausea. Although some people put it down to hormones, and state that it is normal, I believe one reason for it is that it is a sign from the body that we're nutrient deficient in some area and/ or severely dehydrated. Ensuring an adequate intake of the vitamin B range (in liquid form) will help to prevent nausea. Some mothers have success with maca ~ a Peruvian root, which is powdered. Use it in smoothies. Raspberry leaf tea, ginger root tea, peach tea are helpful.

Consider this physical reaction to pregnancy as a reflection of something you're not emotionally expressing. What might you be 'rejecting' about pregnancy that is making you feel sick?

Self reflection

It can be helpful to ask why we might be experiencing pregnancy as a 'sickness'. Many women are troubled by discomfort from eating the wrong foods and drinks ~ in the form of heartburn. The best bet is to avoid spices, fried foods, and soft drinks. Some herbs can be helpful, if taken as a tea.

Extreme tiredness is one symptom of low iron levels. Ensure your diet is rich in dark green leafy vegetables (preferably raw), organic blackstrap molasses, nettles, dried apricots. Ask yourself why you feel drained. Is there something, emotionally, that is stripping your life-force?

You can avoid vaginal and nipple thrush by eliminating sweet and yeasty foods. Limit your sugar consumption, and only have natural sugar ~ in fresh fruit. This will help you avoid gestational diabetes. The more dark leafy green vegetables you include in your diet, the less likely you are to crave sugar-based foods. If you crave sugar, ask yourself "Why do I need extra sweetening? What am I missing emotionally, that I seek in a sweetener? How else can I meet this need for nurturing?"

Calming teas for headaches include chamomile, hops, and peppermint. You may need cranio-sacral or chiropractic sessions. I recommend this for all pregnant and postpartum women, and their babies.

The Birthkeeper's Kitchen

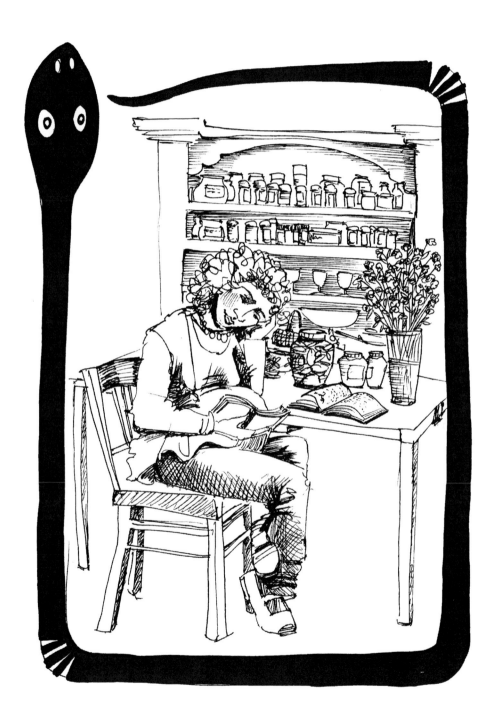

Optimal nutrition is fundamental to self-nurturing. We can self-nurture in many ways, not just through food and drink. How we feed ourselves, and our growing baby, is reflective of how we value ourselves. Our culture teaches as that to self-love is wrong, that it is somehow egotistical. Yet true self-love is the key to loving all of humanity.

So, how do you love yourself? What food choices do you make? Do you seek out foods that you know will nurture your body, or do you reach for something quick and easy and dead, in order to get on with some other activity? Much has been taught over the generations about the four food groups as the basis of good nutrition. We've been led to believe (due to heavy advertising investment by certain industries) that flesh and milk from another animal are vital to our health. Nothing could be further from the truth.

The diet best suited to the human body is a plant-based one, rich in living foods (unprocessed and raw). When we choose to eat anything else, we engage in a dumbing down of both body and soul. You wouldn't put inferior petrol in your car, so why put an inferior fuel into your body? It doesn't make sense, and yet it's what we do in civilised society every day, and for most people, at every meal.

The Birthkeeper becomes aware of her food addictions, and seeks to replace feelings of inadequacy by nurturing herself in ways that are healthful. If she finds herself reaching for a doughnut, she asks herself 'why?'. She will then seek to meet the need for sweetness, or to deaden an emotional pain, in another, healthy way. The Birthkeeper might turn to her journal, and dialogue with the internal angst, or ask her partner for a massage. She might take a long bath, with gentle music, by candle light. The Birthkeeper might meditate. She seeks to keep her feelings conscious. In doing so, she not only heals herself, but avoids her baby learning about addictions before he is even born. Love always brings up anything unlike itself to be healed. When carrying a baby in utero, we are offered a huge opportunity to heal our own gestation, birth and childhood. We can choose to attend to this healing, fully, openly and consciously, or we can run. Many women run to food. Food offers a way of 'stuffing', or suppressing, the feeling. For some women, denial of food is also a way of avoiding feelings. By denying food, we send the message to our self and our baby that we're not worthy.

Learn to find positive ways of nourishing yourself and you'll find life feels more beautiful and radiant. Ensure that your diet is water-rich, that is, filled with raw, living fruits and vegetables.

The way we eat is based on habit. As creatures of habit, we can easily change bad habits and put into place ones which will serve us well. By taking an active interest in your physical vehicle (your body), and providing optimal fuel, you'll quickly discover which foods help you run better, longer, faster.

Wholefood Kitchen Pantry list

Herbal teas
Chamomile
Dandelion
Fennel
Ginger
Ginseng
Lemon Balm
Nettle
Peppermint
Red raspberry
Rosehip
Spearmint
Starflower
Valerian

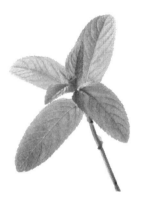

Condiments
Brown rice vinegar
Cider vinegar
Miso
Sauerkraut
Tamari (wheat-free soya sauce)

Herbs & Spices
Aniseed
Basil
Bay leaves
Cardamom
Celery seeds
Chervil
Chives
Cinnamon
Cloves
Coriander
Cumin
Dill
Fenugreek
Garlic
Ginger
Marjoram
Mint
Nutmeg
Oregano
Parsley
Pepper
Rosemary
Saffron
Sage (not while breastfeeding)
Star anise
Tarragon
Thyme
Turmeric
Vanilla

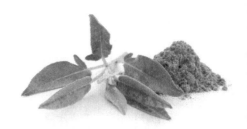

Sweeteners
Agave syrup
Brown rice syrup
Maple syrup
Mirin
Molasses

Seeds
Alfalfa
Flax (Linseed)
Hemp
Pumpkin
Sesame
Sunflower

Sea Vegetables
Arame
Dulse
Hijiki
Kelp
Kombu
Nori sea lettuce
Wakame

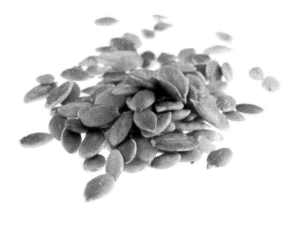

Beans
Adzuki
Borlotti
Broad
Butter
Cannellini
Chickpea
Fava
Flageolet
French
Haricot
Lentil, brown and red
Lima
Mung
Pinto
Soya

Flours
Amaranth, Buckwheat, Chickpea, Gram, Lentil, Oat, Rice, Rye,
Spelt.

Grains
Amaranth
Brown basmati rice
Corn
Kamut
Millet
Oat
Quinoa
Red rice
Spelt
Wild rice

Nuts
Almond
Brazil
Cashew
Coconut
Hazel
Pecan
Pine
Pistachio
Walnut

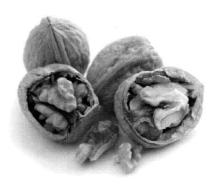

Living Foods

Leafy greens
Beet
Chard
Chicory
Cress
Dandelion (flowers and greens)
Endive
Iceberg
Kale
Gem lettuce
Loose-leaf lettuce
Parsley (flat and curly)
Rocket
Romaine
Sorrel
Swiss chard
Turnip greens
Watercress

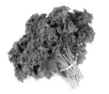

Sprouts
Beansprouts
Alfalfa
Chickpeas
Clover
Mung
Quinoa
Sunflower

Melons
Cantaloupe (rockmelon)
Galia
Honeydew
Watermelon

Fruit
Apple
Apricot
Avocado
Banana
Bilberry
Blackberry
Blackcurrant
Blueberry
Cherry
Cranberry
Damson
Elderberry
Fig
Gooseberry
Grapefruit
Grape
Guava
Fijoa
Kiwi
Kumquat
Lemon
Lime
Loganberry
Loquat
Lychee
Mandarin
Mango
Mulberry
Nectarine
Papaya
Passionfruit
Pawpaw
Peach
Pear
Persimmon
Pineapple
Plum
Pomegranate
Quince

Raspberry
Redcurrant
Rhubarb (really a veg)
Sharon fruit (persimmon)
Starfruit
Strawberry
Tangerine

Dried fruits:
Currant, sultana, raisin; date; apricot,
apple, pear; fig; prune;banana

Vegetables
Artichoke
Asparagus
Aubergine (eggplant)
Avocado
Beetroot
Broccoli
Brussel sprout
Cabbage
Carrot
Cauliflower
Celery
Courgette (zucchini)
Cucumber
Fennel bulb
Globe artichoke
Kohlrabi
Leek
Mangetout
Marrow
Olive
Onion
Oriental leaves
Pak Choi
Parsnip
Pepper (capsicum)
Purple sprouting broccoli
Radish
Red cabbage
Shallot
Spring onion
Squash
Swede
Sweetcorn
Sweet potato
Tomato

Vitamin A
Carrot (raw), spinach, green leafy vegetables, watercress, tomato, red and yellow pepper, mango and dried apricot for cell development, bone and tissue growth, and health of skin and mucus membranes.

Vitamin B complex
Green leafy vegetables, yeast extract, beansprouts, avocado, banana, nuts, mushroom, currant and wholegrain. To avoid depleting your vitamin B levels, you must eliminate stress, alcohol and white products (sugar, flour). The B vitamin range is vital for the development of the nervous system. If you must supplement, opt for vitamin B in liquid form, to avoid the unhealthy fillers often used in tablets.

Vitamin C
Red pepper (capsicum), green leafy vegetables, parsley, kiwi fruit, broccoli, papaya, strawberries, citrus fruits, cantaloupe (rock melon): for the immune system, to help with iron absorption, and for tissue formation.

Vitamin D
The sunshine vitamin ~ needed for strong bones and teeth. It's important to spend at least 20 minutes in full spectrum sunlight each day, regardless of the weather. Don't use sunscreen. Contrary to popular opinion, sunscreens are harmful to the skin, and have been implicated in skin cancers. To avoid sunburn, limit your time in the midday sun, and use shade and a hat/long sleeves.

Vitamin E
Dark green vegetables, tomato, olive oil, tahini, nuts, seeds, avocado, wheat germ oil, oatmeal: needed for circulation, development of cell walls, and tissue growth.

Iodine
Found in kelp, sea vegetables (especially wakame and kombu) and salt. It helps with thyroid function, and is important for energy levels.

Zinc
Found in green vegetables, lentils, almonds, tofu, rice, nuts, seeds, and oats. It's needed for the skeletal and nervous systems, as well as immune function. Lack of zinc leads to a sluggish labour. So, munch on those pumpkin seeds throughout pregnancy!

Iron
Found in blackstrap molasses, dark green leafy vegetables, pumpkin seeds, tofu, prunes, dates, dried apricots, millet and wheat germ. Try drinking stinging nettle tea, too, as it is rich in iron. Iron combines with protein (found in tofu and sunflower seeds, for example) to form haemoglobin. Iron is necessary for healthy energy levels. Avoid taking iron tablets. This is not what your body needs. It does not easily absorb ferrous sulphate. This can lead to miscarriage, constipation, nausea and depleting of vitamin E. Obtain natural iron from your foods, or buy Floradix ~ a natural iron supplement. It's available in good health food shops.

Magnesium
Found in spinach, kelp, brown rice, sesame seeds, prunes, soya beans, cashews, almonds, bananas, honey, bran and leafy green vegetables. Magnesium is needed for muscle action, cellular metabolism and tissue growth. It is believed to help prevent toxaemia in pregnancy.

Rainbow diet for nutrition
When choosing your foods each day, bring to mind a glorious rainbow of colours, and seek to include foods from each colour of the spectrum to 'light up your insides'. There is a reason we were provided with foods of all sorts of colours. This isn't just to make them visually appealing, but because each colour carries its own vibration, and therefore serves a healing purpose when eaten. Always seek the ripest, freshest fruits, vegetables, nuts and seeds.

Energy vibration of food
Living foods contain enzymes, considered to be an invisible energy field. These life-force elements are vital to our good health and well-being. Processed foods are devoid of living enzymes. When our diet lacks them, we miss out on this life-force, and feel sluggish as a result.

Enzymes give our body the message that the food we're eating is partially-digested, so our digestive forces don't have to work so hard. Culturally, the feeling of tiredness after eating cooked food is considered normal. Try having a week eating nothing but foods rich in enzymes, and you'll discover that being sluggish, fatigued and tired are not how we were designed to be.

Organic

Proponents of chemically-based agriculture like to suggest that their produce is no different in nutrition or taste to organically-grown food. Certainly, those people who'd rather not spend their money on organic food would like to hope those proponents are right. Think about this: plants and animals, like us, are living, breathing creatures. If you were regularly coated in all sorts of toxic chemicals, do you think that your skin (which is highly porous) wouldn't absorb those poisons? Would you flourish and be the best you could be in such an environment?

Chemicals used in agriculture and in animal food not only poison the end product, but cause untold damage to soil, air and water. When we eat organic and/or wild-crafted foods, we're saying yes to our body, to our children and to the environment. The same can never be said for conventional agriculture. People often suggest that because toxins are now being found in breast milk, women should start feeding their babies formula! If the toxins are in breast milk, then they will be in your body when you conceive and gestate your baby. If you are concerned about chemicals and pesticides, then take action: eat only organic or wildcrafted foods.

Nutrition and tribal women

My mother's reason for becoming vegetarian was that she'd read in her spiritual studies that vegetarian women tended to have an easier time in childbirth. This is true for menstruation, as well. Unlike Westerners, tribal cultures tend not to overeat, and they don't indulge in gluttony or consume excess calories. Likewise, their diet does not consist of overly fatty foods.

Regardless of whether a particular culture is vegetarian or not, pregnant women in tribes reduce or eliminate meat altogether in pregnancy.

Many tribes felt that meat consumption was linked to difficulty in birth. As well as restricting flesh, animal milk was also forbidden.

Clearly, artificial sweeteners were not present in tribal cultures, either. It is true, however, that early people had access to honey and sugar cane, but these were excluded from the pregnant tribal woman's diet. Interestingly, salt was also forbidden, both in pregnancy and after birth.

Each culture was aware of the local foods which were not suitable for pregnancy, such as hot, spicy or unripe.

As far back as 1932, Grantly Dick-Read was advocating a vegetarian diet, saying that vegetarians "generally have less trouble with pregnancy and labour than those who are heavy meat eaters". Vegetarian, in this case, means someone who primarily eats fruits, vegetables, nuts and seeds, rather than a grain-based diet.

Vibrational Allies

Flower Essences have been used for many years to treat the emotional conditions common to human life. They are considered as a medicine for the soul, because they bring us into touch with our true, magnificent self. Essences are also made from vibrational infusions of gems, animals (no animal is used or harmed), and environment. Essences for use in pregnancy and childbirth have been well researched.

Pear
Pear essence is helpful for women who fear losing control in birth. It brings an inner calm. It's also well known to practitioners as the maternal essence, and promotes breastfeeding.

Starflower
Starflower essence is a breast milk promoter, but just as importantly, brings joy to the heart, and gladdens the mind. It's known for bringing confidence and courage, especially through difficult life circumstances. It can also help a pregnant mother bond with her baby in utero. Consider it for helping with mourning following a miscarriage or stillbirth.

Bougainvillea
Bougainvillea is an essence for the inner child. When taken, it helps us tune into our unborn child. Consider this essence if your baby is breech. It can help the baby to feel safe about presenting head first.

Star of Bethlehem
Used in Bach's Rescue Remedy, this essence is for shock, terror and trauma. It's wonderful for helping a birthing woman integrate all her feelings about birth. Consider it, too, in the case of a traumatic birth.

Self-heal
This is the essence for activating your inner healer. It's particularly good for helping your body absorb nutrients from your food while pregnant, as well as stimulating the immune system.

Dandelion

Use this essence if you need help to honour and understand your instincts and intuition, especially during pregnancy, labour and birth. It's very useful in the last stage of labour, when a woman is having trouble 'letting go'.

Pomegranate

This essence is for bringing out one's femininity, and helps you to feel confident in your femaleness during pregnancy and birth.

Chamomile
This is useful for grounding one's self in birth, as it brings calmness and a sense of knowing where you are. Regardless of how the birth is progressing, this essence allows for confidence and calm.

Olive
Olive essence is for when you feel you can't go on: exhaustion in mind and body. It's very helpful for lack of sleep after birth.

Elm
Elm essence suits those mothers who feel completely overwhelmed by parenting and the sheer responsibility of caring for another human being.

Hornbeam
This is for apathy: when you can't be bothered even brushing your hair or teeth.

Oak
For the workaholic-mother, who doesn't slow down in her mothering to nurture herself ~ the mother who keeps going until she's utterly exhausted/driven on by responsibility.

Following the birth of your baby, the following essences may be of use:

Starflower
For promoting breast milk and finding the instinct to nurture your child.

Walnut
This is excellent for any change in life: puberty, teething, exams, birth, house move, etc. Dads and siblings should also consider taking this essence. Add a few drops to a water spray bottle, and spray around the house; or add a couple of drops to a glass of water.

Gorse
Consider this essence if you're feeling the post-partum blues.

Other essences to consider:

Fig
Use this essence to prepare for conception and pregnancy.

Watermelon
Perfect for use before and after conception. It's useful for relieving any emotional stress in pregnancy. It releases breast milk.

Hairy Butterwort
This Alaskan flower essence helps us to be conscious during the transition stage of labour and birth.

Cauliflower
This is used both for helping the soul adjust to arriving Earthside, and also for releasing the trauma of coming to Earth. It's suitable for the baby. Rub a drop on their ankle.

Keurtjie
This South African essence is for increasing the ability to nurture, and at the same time, to feel nurtured. Fathers will find this useful too, for feelings of post-natal depression they may be experiencing.

Essential Oils

Many maternity units in Western society are starting to recognise the science of Aromatherapy, and are incorporating the use of essential oils into their maternity practice.

Regardless of your choice of birth place, consider bringing oils into your birthing room. Studies show that foetal and maternal stress can be eased when mothers are given an aromatherapy massage in labour.

What you will need:
[] A dark coloured glass bottle/s for storing your oil.

[] A carrier oil, such as almond or grape seed.

[] Essential oils (ensure these really are essential oils, and not synthetic fragrances).

[] Cloths, if using as a compress.

The only oils to use for aromatherapy are those labelled as therapeutic. These are botanically sourced and do not contain any additives, nor have they had chemicals used in the distillation process. They are steamed under intense pressure, to guarantee completeness. You must ensure the highest grade oils for use as a healing agent.

Some aromatherapists have worried that there are oils which shouldn't be used in pregnancy because they are emmenagogic, which means they can bring on the menstrual cycle. However, research by pharmacologist Tony Balacs shows otherwise. He states that during pregnancy they don't act as an abortifacient.

There are certain oils, however, which must be avoided in pregnancy. These are: ajowan, aniseed, basil, bitter almond, cornmint, fennel, hyssop, mugwort, oregano, parsley seed, pennyroyal, sage, sweet birch, sweet marjoram, transy, tarragon, thyme, bay leaf, wild thyme, wintergreen, wormseed and wormwood.

To use:
Massage ~ Use 10 drops of essential oil to 2 ounces of base oil (sweet almond or grapeseed).

Bath ~ Use 5 drops of essential oil in your bath. Mix with your hand before entering the water, to ensure the oil has spread sufficiently.

Compress ~ Add 3 drops of oil to a bowl of water of desired temperature. Soak a face cloth in the water, and then wring out. Place it on the desired part of the body.

Inhalation ~ If you're using an oil burner, use 3 drops in water.

Recommended essential oils for pregnancy:
Neroli (relieves anxiety)
Bergamot (releases fears and anxiety)
Rose (allows calm, and dispels fears)
Frankincense (calming)
Lavender (promotes pain relief, and offers relaxation in labour)
Jasmine (useful for strengthening contractions)

Homeopathic Remedies
Homeopathy is safe, gentle yet powerful, and can be used by everyone. It is based on the idea of like curing like. Each remedy works on a vibrational level. If this modality of healing resonates with you, it is worth consulting a professional homeopath and exploring it further.

Anaemia
Ferrum Met tissue salt.
Ferrum Phos tissue salt.

Backache
Bellis: Pubis bone splits.
Hypericum: Coccyx pain.
Oak: Affinity with the spine, helps strengthen spine.
Sepia: Lower back, dragging down pains.

Birth Trauma
Caesium & Carbo veg: Collapsed body, baby blue with breathing difficulties.
Obsidian: For any kind of crushing; traumatic forceps delivery.

Contractions
Arnica: Helps support the body to do what it needs to do.
Silver birch: Contractions are too fast, and are painful to cope with.

Kidney Support
Apis Mel: Affinity with kidneys, oedema, water retention.
Hazel: For water balance, and to support kidneys in general.
Sandalwood: For pre-eclampsia.

Malpresentation of a baby
Pulsatillia or Peridot: For a breech presenting baby.

Morning Sickness
Ipecac: Persistent nausea with/without vomiting, where the mother is no better for vomiting or eating.

Nux Vom: Irritability, hypersensitive to noise, lights, people, smells.
Sepia: can't be bothered to do anything, vomits in the afternoon.
Feels better for eating.
Blue: Nausea with anxiety; helps the mother surrender to her pregnancy.
Sandalwood: Calming effect. Protection during birth. Brings the new soul into consciousness.

Pain relief during labour
Arnica, calendula, bellis: If the mother tears during birth.

Piles
Aesculus: Affinity with the pelvis, lower back. Constipation and piles. Congestion.
Hamamelis: Towards end of pregnancy. After childbirth. Profuse bleeding.

Remedies for pregnancy
Almond: Stimulation of the baby's brain. Security and integration aspect of mother and baby.

Remedies for newborn
Aconite: Nervous, fearful baby; quick birth.
Arnica: Traumatic birth.

Scans
Obsidian: Protection of the foetus before and after the scan.
Rainbow: Combats radiation, removes negative energy.

Threatened Miscarriage
Apple tree: Miscarriage due to the baby not quite being present in the developing physical body. The mother being in a vulnerable emotional state.
Emerald: Repeated miscarriages in the 3rd month of pregnancy.

Herbs

Well before the rise of professional midwifery, women were aware of how herbal knowledge could bring great benefits to pregnancy and birth. If you intend to use herbs, in almost all cases it is best to grow them yourself or find wild ones away from pollution and pesticides. If purchasing them, avoid synthetic-based herbs, and opt for tinctures or dried leaves, roots, seeds or flowers for teas. In all cases, opt for organically-grown or wildcrafted herbs from reputable herb farms.

Red raspberry leaf tea

One of the most well-known herbal tonics is the tea made from leaves of the Red Raspberry. It has been documented as a uterine stimulant for thousands of years. Safely drunk throughout pregnancy, this herb helps the uterus to tone up in preparation for birth. It helps to avoid postpartum bleeding, as well as returning the uterus to pre-pregnancy size. Raspberry leaves are high in iron, and are especially suitable for preventing iron deficiency (anaemia).

Black cohosh

Used by Native American Indians to great effect, it makes labour stronger and regulates contractions. Do not use it in capsule form. Seek out a tincture. Do not use if you suffer from blood clotting or anaemia. Take 5 – 10 drops of the tincture every half hour. Stop when labour starts. Do not use for more than a 24 hour period.

Blue cohosh: as above, but also to strengthen the uterus while it is contracting. Take 10 -15 drops every hour.

Nettles

Never scoff at these weeds, for nettles are packed with nutrients, most notably iron, folic acid and calcium. Women who regularly consume nettles find they prevent varicose veins, retained fluid, and support the adrenal system, kidneys, and promote breast milk. Nettles can be used in cooking. Treat as spinach, and use in familiar dishes like lasagne. Don't worry about the sting in the leaves; it goes during cooking. It's best to pick nettles in Spring and Summer.

If you have access to plenty of nettles which have been grown away from pollution etc., then harvest a bunch to freeze for use in the winter.

Dandelion Roots
As a tea, this root relieves constipation and brings healing support to the liver. It contains good amounts of calcium and iron. If you have access to fresh dandelion leaves, add them to salads or home-made juices, as they're rich in vitamin A. Try drinking dandelion tea, as it's high in potassium.

Alfalfa
Rich in vitamin K (essential for blood clotting), chlorophyll, and many trace minerals, this is worth having as a food or tea in the last trimester of pregnancy. It also increases breast milk.

Oats
Considered a herbal medicine, oat is also high in calcium, as well as magnesium ~ so vital for the nervous system, as well as essential for the healthy building of bones. You can choose to have oats for breakfast (avoid sugar, and use agave syrup, to sweeten, and add rice milk). Oatstraw tea is also available.

Herbs don't just work on the physical body, but also help to calm our emotions and ease any pain that may surface as a result of our fears.

If you're looking for a herb to ease pain, consider chamomile ~ as it helps by relieving the built-up tension in the body. Crampbark is well known for getting rid of afterbirth pains. If you've got catnip growing in the garden, remember, it's not just for your cat. It helps to calm and relax humans, too.

Before birth, you might like to make up a mixture for a sooth-ing birth massage oil. This will ease pain, relax muscles, soothe and soften the perineum, and ease any burning sensation caused from tension. Add lavender, rose and chamomile to a base of sweet al-mond oil. A few drops of each oil per ½ litre of base oil is more than enough.

Postpartum haemorrhage

Midwives worth their salt always keep the tincture of Shepherd's Purse with them in case of an emergency. It is the number one herb to stop a postpartum bleed.

Perineal Care

Use a shallow bath after birth if you wish to support the perineum. Use herbs of Shepherd's Purse, Yarrow, Garlic, Witch Hazel and Uva Ursi. These will reduce swelling and heal tears. You can also put this mixture into a spray bottle to soothe you while urinating.

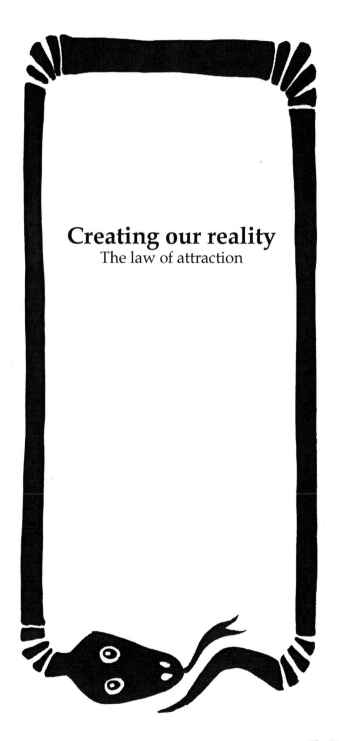

Creating our reality
The law of attraction

Birthing with medical attendants in the room often means that birth is purely a physical event: women are usually treated in a way that doesn't take into account their whole being ~ mind, body and soul. A holistic birth acknowledges that we are spiritual beings in a physical (human) body, with complex needs ~ emotional, psychological, sexual and spiritual. Given our true nature, we have to question the place of medical machines and medically-minded people observing and monitoring what is essentially a sacred, sexual experience. We have to question their impact on our sensitive self.

The worst device in a labour room is the clock on the wall. In hospital, the medically-based midwives decide how long your labour should be, and when to give you drugs to make things move along. Birthing drugs speed labour up, and often make it intense or painful. It becomes a vicious circle where the mum then pleads for more drugs, of a different sort, to help her get through birth. These cross the placenta to the baby, which slows his start in life. A drugged birth inhibits the mother from fully accessing her birth and bonding hormones. It's quite common for women to close down to birthing, and 'need' a caesarean. Her whole mammalian way of being has been interrupted. Shutting down her body (through fear) is a way of ensuring her baby is kept safe. Her body is acting instinctively, and any woman who has experienced this in her birth should NOT feel guilty or ashamed.

A woman's mammalian brain isn't to know that she and her baby are going to be in far more danger: that a knife is going to go dangerously close to her baby. Many babies have been scarred for life due to meeting a scalpel at birth. Regardless of whether we have a DIY unobserved homebirth, a midwife-attended homebirth, or have our baby delivered in hospital, each of us is responsible for the birth of our baby.

It's simply not possible for a doctor or midwife to be responsible for your birth. We may think that having a Paid Paranoid tending our birth will help if there are complications; however, we must be mindful that complications don't 'just' happen. They happen for a reason ~ the reason being, that they were 'caused'. The Birthkeeper knows how to prevent such complications. She does so by avoiding many standard procedures, by knowing she has a choice, and that her beautiful birth outcome manifests by her listening to her inner voice, rather than an external one.

The Birthkeeper takes conscious responsibility by making a commitment to having a peaceful and healthy pregnancy, and knowing that no-one else is responsible for how she eats, thinks, exercises and acts. We're never more open ~ physically, psychically or emotionally ~ than when we're giving birth. For this reason alone, being safe within the walls of our own home, in the company of those we love, is the only place we should give birth if we want to respect and revere our mammalian needs. An unobtrusive midwife still brings her own baggage with her, and can never truly see beyond the boundaries around the birthing woman. She (or he) can be the most well-meaning, beautiful, wise, devoted, kind midwife in the world, but she still can not access a woman's innermost self, and nor should she try.

The best midwife is one who sits on her hands, listening quietly from another room. Such a midwife listens with her heart, and knows where a woman is at in labour by the sounds she is making. A spiritual midwife has no need to do internal examinations or to take blood pressure. Such midwives are few and far between. If you invite a midwife to your birth, ask about her birthing history ~ of birthing her own babies and the births she has attended. How many of her women birthed ecstatically? How many ended up as 'birth rape'? Her honest answers will let you know what her beliefs are about birth.

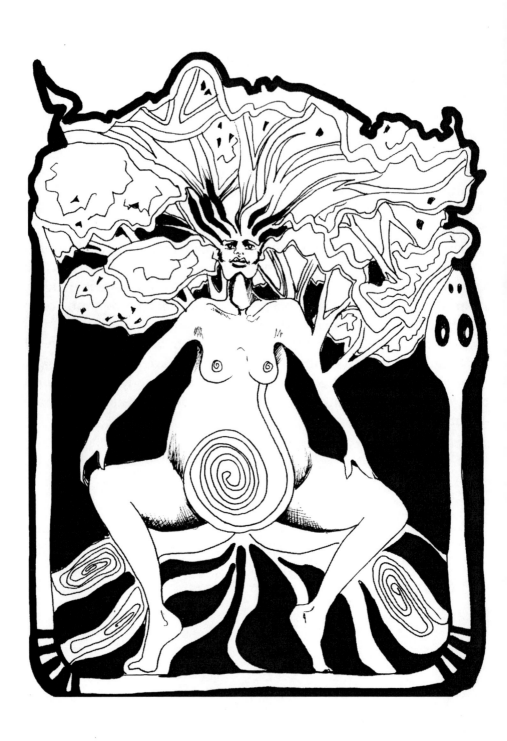

Equipment

Many women planning an unassisted birth have asked me what equipment they'll need. Essentially, you're planning for a home-birth, but with the awareness that the midwife will not be arriving with her tool kit. Your tool kit is your body and your intuition. Your inner eyes and ears will guide you through this process. By the time you've reached birth, you'll have developed a deep awareness and the ability to listen to the still, small voice within. In addition to this, I recommend:

Your thinking

The most fundamental difference between our ancient tribal sisters and modern birthing women is that our ancestresses fully trusted their body to birth easily and effortlessly. They knew their body was designed to give birth. A modern birthing woman often expects to have her baby delivered from her, and has bought into the belief that birth is dangerous.

Humans are made of water. We start our lives made up of 90% water, by midlife this is nearer 70%, and by old age, it's down to 50%. Water, as studied by Masuro Emoto, is shown to hold memories. His fascinating works have enthralled millions of people throughout the world.

Given that we are primarily made of water, and that we are impacted by things such as the Moon's cycle, it makes sense that what we think and feel will magnetise certain events into our lives. Like Emoto's water crystals, which react to words such as love, hate, anger, fear, joy, etc., our body's electromagnetic nature is that we have an intense desire to manifest our feelings and thoughts into our reality. Our thoughts become manifest, and the stronger the thought, the more quickly it materialises. Physicists have proven what author Richard Bach says, "We magnetise into our lives whatever we hold in our thought." And of course, knowing what we know about water, this makes perfect sense. As living, vibrant, mostly-water beings, we do magnetise what we're thinking or feeling. The most supportive thing a birthing woman can do for her self is to release the cultural thoughts that birth is 'dangerous, deadly and painful'. This is vital for all women, regardless of whether they choose to birth alone, or with midwives, machines and men in attendance.

Changing our thoughts and subconscious beliefs can be done in various ways, such as through affirmations, prayer, meditation, journaling, Breathwork, EFT (emotional freedom technique), chiropractic or cranio-sacral therapy ~ to release blockages, etc. If using affirmations, it is important to write and say them in the present tense (acting as if), and to keep them positive. For example, if you were to affirm "I don't want a painful birth" your subconscious would hear the part about "painful birth", and like a dutiful servant would deliver that to you. Rather, you would say "I enjoy an easy birthing". Affirmation examples include:

I birth easily and effortlessly
I love giving birth
I am made to birth beautifully
Birth is pleasurable
I am safe giving birth
My baby is safe being born
My baby loves being born
I am loved, loving and lovable
I am grateful for the ability to give birth naturally and ecstatically to my baby
My body opens to birth easily
My baby is in the optimal foetal position for an easy vaginal birth

You could also write words on paper, and place them under a glass of spring water for a while before drinking it. Suggested words include: beautiful birth; bliss; love and gratitude; health; peace; surrender; trust; safe.

Prayer

Many people use prayer as a way of begging for something. That is certainly what mainstream religion would teach us. I prefer to see prayer as a dialogue between the one praying and the Divine, not based on grovelling, but gratitude.

My conversations with the Universe are one of appreciation ~ of knowing that I have everything I need at all times. If I ever feel the need to find a solution to something, rather than asking to 'have it fixed up', I ask that I be shown a way to clear whatever blocks I have about the situation.

Meditation

As already stated, meditation helps to find the calm and peace which always exists within us. Meditation, whether it includes finding a gap in the mind-space, gently chanting a mantra, or conscious relaxation, offers a place and space to still the outside world, and step away from our culture's invisible force field.

If at all possible, meditate outside, in Nature, as the Earth's frequency is conducive to the meditative state.

A Living Meditation is one where you are consciously present in every moment: being aware that you are the observer of your life. This is as relevant if taking a walk, sitting still, washing the dishes or changing your baby's nappy.

Warm room

It's important for mother and babe to be warm after birth. If it isn't possible to warm the room, then it's vital for warmth to be available through hot water bottles and blankets. The providing of warmth after birth is common in all birthing cultures.

Oils for massage

It can be very comforting for the labouring woman to receive massages during or between contractions. Use a base of almond or grape seed oil, then add a desired essential oil. Check that it is suitable for pregnancy. Lavender is particularly soothing. Ensure that the oil has been gently warmed.

Catching your baby

The female body is designed so that the birthing mother will catch her own baby, rather than have it delivered from her. Nature ordained that we would reach forward and bring our baby up, from the vagina, and into our arms. Physiologically, this means the direct, upward motion of the baby brings him/her up over the bone at the front of the mother's pelvis. By doing so, tearing the perineum (so common in modern births) is prevented.

Birth ball (optional)

Some women enjoy having a birthing ball to lean on during labour. As with any birthing prop, remember to keep upright or on all fours.

Birth pool

Highly recommended, even if you don't wish to birth in water. Labouring in water allows you to work with buoyancy, rather than gravity. Warm water helps a woman ease into the experience of labour. It has the added benefit of really softening the perineum, so that it relaxes, and accommodates the baby's head easily. For the baby, this is the ideal transition from watery womb life to landing into a gravity-ruled world. It is far too easy to underestimate or ignore how shocking it is for a newborn to arrive into air and gravity. Birth in water makes the arrival Earthside so much gentler.

Music

If you wish to play music during labour or birth, choose something positive and uplifting, which is soothing, relaxing and nurturing. This isn't a time for rock music or something jarring to the senses! You need to slow your heartbeat, not to be on an unnatural adrenalin rush.

Vibrational essences

Some women utilise Nature's medicine cabinet to support their birthing journey. These natural vibrational remedies work on an emotional level.

Cloth re-usable menstrual pads

Cloth menstrual pads are washable, therefore reusable over and over again, and avoid toxic chemicals from disposable pads and tampons going near your vagina, not to mention pollution in landfills and seas. You'll need menstrual products to catch your lochia (post birth blood loss) ~ some women have a discharge for up to six weeks. Drink red raspberry leaf tea to help contract the uterus to its pre-birth size, as well as putting babe straight to your breast.

T-shirt, nightdress

If you feel so inclined, wear some loose clothing, like a t-shirt or nightdress. Some women find any clothing a complete hindrance to pleasurable birthing.

Blankets

Our temperature fluctuates during labour, so access to blankets is important. They're useful after birth as well.

Source of heating
Always have a back up source available for mother and child ~ such as a heater, open fire, hot water bottle.

Beverages and snacks
Pure spring water
Lemon and honey/agave
Fresh fruit and vegetable juices
Raspberry leaf tea iceblocks with agave syrup
Easy to eat, soft, ripe fruit, such as berries
Vegetables and dip
Crackers ~ something simple like oat or rice crackers are best, and they're less exhausting on the digestive system than wheat crackers.

Birth Companions
Who have you invited to your birth? Every person in attendance brings their beliefs (positive or negative) about birth and death into the birthing room. It's your responsibility, as a birthing mother, to ensure that whoever is in your birthing space is free of their fears, and that they trust birth as a natural part of life.

Hand mirror
Some women like to have a hand mirror available in case they want to see the baby's head as it crowns. Other mothers are happy to have it remembered as an entirely sensual experience, i.e., feeling the head with their hand.

Candles
Candles are best for low lighting. Be aware that your baby is coming from quite a dark place into a well-lit world. Use beeswax or plant-based candles, and avoid petrochemical ones.

Camera/video
If you choose to film your birth in any way, try to ensure it is done in a non-obtrusive way. These tools act as another set of eyes, and the observation of these pieces of technology can hinder labour as much as having the wrong person in the birthing room. Be aware that some cameras are noisy, and can be intrusive in this way, too.

Vitamin K

Make an informed decision about whether you want your baby to have vitamin K after the birth. Those in the medical profession give the injection as routine, in order to protect against haemorrhagic disease of the newborn (HDN) ~ most often caused by birth trauma resulting from medically-managed births. The condition is extremely rare. Estimates suggest that it causes death or serious injury in approximately 1 in 10,000 babies. The main concerns with vitamin K are that babies have low levels of it at birth; however, this doesn't mean that it's wrong for them to have low levels. Nature had her own reasons for a baby having different vitamin K levels to her parents. If you're concerned about vitamin K, but want to avoid synthetic products going into your baby, then ensure your maternal diet is rich in vitamin K. And remember, this vitamin is in breast milk, so get your baby onto the breast straight after birth. Intravenous vitamin K has been linked to childhood leukaemia.

Skin products

Avoid putting any products (that you wouldn't eat) onto your baby's skin. A baby's sense of smell is extremely sensitive. Avoid deodorants, perfumes and strong shampoos. Let your baby enjoy your natural body smells. This is really important for bonding.

First breath

When I was a baby, it was routine for newborns to be held upside down by their feet, and for the doctor to administer a slap across the buttocks. Why? It was to ensure that the baby took its first breath. Most people were led to believe that the cry which then followed was of benefit to the baby and showed everyone he or she had a good set of healthy lungs. We've slowly moved away from such a barbaric practice and recognise both the trauma of such crying, and the unnecessary act of hitting. A newborn need only be massaged or rubbed gently by her mother in order to stimulate breathing.

Our tribal ancestresses would clear the baby's mouth of mucus by using their finger. In some cultures, it was normal to either bathe the baby in cold water, or sprinkle with cold water, to initiate healthy breathing, before being bathed in warm water.

Many cultures around the world
report an easy delivery
of the placenta at birth.
Unlike modern births,
the placenta is never
tugged or pulled at.

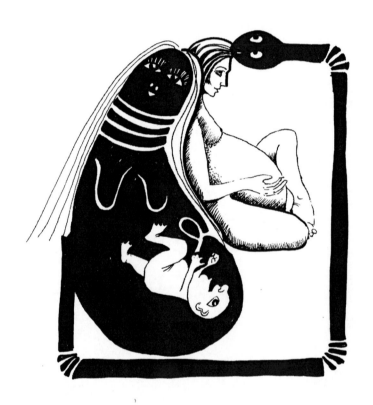

Premature babies

The most important need of a baby who has been born early, is that of warmth. Although prematurity was rare in ancient cultures, they did have ways of providing the necessary warmth to an early arrival baby. Most tribes used soft feathers. One culture, the Basongye of Zaire, would give the baby a steam bath for a few moments. They would do this about six times a day for a week.

The best care we can give our modern premature babies is to remove them from their incubators and place them under their mother's shirt. It's absolutely vital that a premature baby gets this warmth and *heart to heart* intensive care.

Breathing during labour

Our tribal ancestresses also had an innate understanding of the use of breath throughout labour and birth. Most significant of all, perhaps, is that most of these women didn't yell out during birth.

Perineum

Epidurals and vaginal tears are common in Western culture, yet tribal women supported the perineum in birth through various natural means. Often, the birthing woman would sit (knees flexed) over sand which was covered by an animal skin. By doing so, she could allow the sand to mould against her perineum. Modern women need not sit on sand and animal skins, but can birth in water, which acts as a beautiful support to the perineal tissues.

Our ancestresses often bathed or steamed the perineum; and some women softened the flesh with an oil-based lubricant ~ regularly massaging this area during pregnancy.

Malpresentation

Western women routinely face caesarean if their baby is presenting as breech or transverse. It would seem that because massage was so commonly used in tribal cultures, malpresentation was uncommon. According to Joseph Chilton Pearce, in Evolution's End, the female body is designed for birth to take an average of 20 minutes (including labour). It makes sense then that our body should have the easiest presentation possible.

The two ways of dealing with malpresentation were to turn the baby, either externally (cephalic) or internally (podalic). Throughout the world's oldest societies, cephalic was the more commonly used technique, and pregnant women were routinely massaged during pregnancy. The podalic version was rare, and was always used as a last minute technique.

Birth position

The most common birth position for our ancestresses was squatting. Most Western women find this position difficult because they've not had adequate exercise to strengthen their leg muscles. By squatting, the birthing woman is able to widen the birth canal. Squatting, kneeling or sitting allows a birthing woman the greatest control over her experience.

A Western woman who has her feet up in stirrups, or is forced to lie on her back, is in the worst possible position for giving birth, and will almost certainly end up being 'delivered' of her baby. It's no surprise that this position was brought about in the late 1600s by an obstetrician. Obstetrician is derived from the root word, obstare ~ which means: to stand in the way.

In very simple terms, if you imagine giving birth as requiring the same force of gravity as doing a poo, then you can see how insane lying on your back really is. Of course, using a toilet was not Nature's intention either. If you've ever been lucky enough to go to the loo naturally, that is, squatting on the ground, you'll have discovered how much easier it is to release all faecal matter in one go ~ quickly, easily and without strain.

After childbirth

Most modern women are confined to hospital beds immediately after birth. Tribal women stand up straight after birth, and many would do a fair bit of walking as this would prevent haemorrhage. Aside from exercise, ancient women also had their own ways of cleaning themselves up after birth. Some tribes who lived near sea water would enter, and clean themselves thoroughly with the salt water. Often they'd take a lump of moss or something similar to help in the cleaning process. The water wasn't only for cleaning, but to rejuvenate the circulatory system, as the water was almost always cold. One particular tribe, from Oceania, the Marquesans, enjoyed sexual intercourse straight after birth.

They would do this in a stream, and found it to be therapeutic. Cultures which were not based near moving water had other methods of cooling the birthing mother, such as applying fresh sage to her face. *Foetus Ejection Reflex:* If there's one thing most people could tell you about birth (regardless of whether they've had children), it's that you'll need someone (doctor, midwife, ambulance driver or husband) to tell you when to push. This is reinforced in every television programme and movie depicting birth. The idea that you have to force the baby out of your birth canal through unbelievable effort, is one of the biggest birthing myths which exists. Foetus ejection reflex is the body's way of ensuring your baby comes out. This is a reflex, which means it happens of its own accord and doesn't need any 'coaching'. Women who've birthed on their own, without any interference, will tell you that the urge to push just came over them and that they didn't have to do anything to help it along.

The cord and the placenta

If Mother Nature had intended the cord and placenta of a human to be separated straight after birth, She'd have designed a way for the separation to happen without our intervention, or given us the teeth of a carnivore. There are many reasons why we should not attempt to artificially separate the relationship between the placenta (the baby's other mother, as it is a source of nourishment for nine months), the cord and the baby. Transfusion takes place between the placenta and baby after birth. Cord blood is vital for the long term health of the baby, and the cord shouldn't be prematurely cut. Some people choose to wait till the cord stops pulsing, however this isn't the only indication of the life force being transferred. Interestingly, our tribal sisters approached the cord in different ways, depending on their customs. Many cultures around the world report an easy delivery of placenta at birth. Unlike modern births, the placenta is never tugged or pulled at. In any case where it may need helping along, massage is implemented. Almost always, massage works to bring on placental delivery. In the rare cases where this doesn't work, finding ways to cause a woman's abdominal muscles to contract (through gagging, blowing or sneezing) suffice. Some cultures, such as that of the Moroccans, traditionally use heat. They soak the severed end of the cord in oil which had been heated. The placenta falls out within a few minutes.

Heat is also used by the Mexicans, who place a hot tortilla on the mother's side. The Cahuilla and Benua-Jakun encourage the mother to stand over a fire. Probably one of the most revealing and beautiful aspects of tribal cultures is that of patience. In all but the rarest of circumstances, they know that by being patient, all births will end well.

By far the most common and effective way to bring down the placenta is by encouraging the newborn to nurse straight after birth. Breastfeeding stimulates the hormone oxytocin, which helps to contract the uterus. This also contracts the small blood vessels where the placenta joins the uterus, and helps to stop bleeding becoming excessive.

Tribal cultures, for the most part, do not cut the cord before the placenta is expelled. The major difference between traditional cord cutting and modern cord cutting is that tribal cultures do not use metal. Various instruments were used, such as a sharp shell or blunt glass. Commonly, something like thread or string would be used. It is believed that metal has a negative effect on human flesh.

If you do wish to cut the cord, leave it for at least a few hours if at all possible. The placenta can be wrapped in a re-usable nappy, and tucked up right beside you and the baby. Once cut, dress the cord stump with New Zealand Manuka honey. It has unique anti-bacterial properties, which prevent infection. You could also dab lavender or tea-tree oil on the stubbed end. Avoid using plastic pegs, and use soft string, instead, to tie off the cord. Remember, it is a wound ~ physical, emotional and spiritual.

If you experience intensely painful contractions in the days after birth, Motherwort tincture is very beneficial. It's always better for you and your baby to opt for natural products rather than to resort to synthetic pain relief.

Lotus Born

Psychics who have tuned into newborn babies have concluded that when the cord remains uncut it allows the baby to come fully Earthside into his body. The moment at which the cord naturally breaks is the time the baby has fully arrived. In my own experience of cord cutting, we left Bethany's cord for quite some time ~ until well after it had stopped pulsating: about half an hour. Until the moment we cut the cord, she hadn't made a peep, but quietly observed her parents and her surroundings. As soon as our midwife cut the cord, Bethany cried. She was clearly very distressed by it, even though she was in my arms, in the warmth of the birthing pool.

Women whose children have had a lotus birth report that their children are very calm and centred. Hopefully such anecdotal stories will gather respect and support from the fields of science and psychology before too long.

Many parents agree that their lotus birthed baby retained a sense of connectedness ~ contentment.

If you choose a lotus birth, simply wrap the placenta in a cotton nappy and keep it close to the baby. Some mothers sprinkle salt or lavender oil on the placenta, daily. Initially, you might like to place the placenta in a colander, on top of a large bowl, to drain the blood and wash off any clots.

Keep sprinkling it with lavender each day. When the cord dries and breaks off, after a few days, you might like to plant the placenta under a tree, for example, at your baby's Naming Ceremony.

I'm always intrigued by how our own experience of being birthed influences our view of how we support other mothers and babies in their birth process. During rebirthing and primal therapy, people have relived the trauma and pain not only of birth, but of having the cord cut. If we're unwilling to listen to our babies, perhaps we might take notice of the messages from adults who've undergone hypnosis.

Clearing out psychic pollution

Psychic pollution exists all around us in Culture's invisible field. We're born into it, despite the intention of our parents. Our materialistic culture, which at best, grasps at a saccharine spirituality, doesn't encourage self-love, conscious awareness and personal empowerment. Indeed, efforts are constantly made to ensure we don't think for ourselves, and don't find answers to our soul's questions and deep yearnings.

One of the best ways for culture to control people is by beginning at birth, with women and their babies. Having our primal instincts controlled so that we can't birth according to our mammalian needs, immediately puts us into the arena of being dependent on others to save us from the 'faults' of Nature. We're taught at every turn that Nature can't be trusted, and we're given alternatives: such as formula instead of breast milk; a cot/crib instead of a mother's arms; school instead of learning from life.

Many years ago, in New Zealand, I had the pleasure and privilege of working for a well-known self-hypnosis teacher. After he taught people self-hypnosis, I would lead follow-up workshops. People from all walks of life learnt this invaluable skill, including leading sportspeople. Nobody doubts that such skills, which include creative visualisation and affirmations, help sports men and women to achieve their aims. Increasingly, this skill has been used in the field of childbirth. If the power of the mind is considered 'proven' in the field of sports, then we can only assume it is also relevant to how we visualise our birth 'performance'. What we visualise, imagine, affirm and think about in relation to our pregnancy, birth and parenting is what will manifest physically for us, and will bring up our fears. It's important to address and clear these before birth. We need to be aware of the people around us at birth, and what beliefs they bring with them.

The boundaries at birth

There is no moment in life when a woman is more physically, and spiritually, open than when her baby is crowning. At this moment, between Spiritside and the baby's entry Earthside, the mother straddles two worlds. It is rarely considered, in prenatal education and support, how a woman's childhood experiences may impact on how she gives birth.

Sexual abuse in childhood is commonplace, with as many as one in four girls being inappropriately touched or raped (and the degrees of abuse between those two ends). It's also just as common for girls to grow into women who never share their 'secret'. Unless we resolve our feelings of hurt, betrayal, confusion, guilt and fear, we risk bringing them to light in the birthing room when our psychic wounds come up for healing. Personally, I found that choosing to birth at home, away from unknown men in masks, with violating tools, enabled me to take charge of my sexual self at birth. The birthing pool created a physical barrier around me during my emergence into that open expression of sexuality.

What often happens, for a woman who's experienced abuse in childhood, is that she subconsciously recreates the violation by having a birth where she is 'raped' through use of ventouse, forceps or episiotomy, or, through hands doing internal exams.

You can seek professional support, or choose to work through your pain and memories on your own or with your life partner. I have always found journaling very helpful in writing down fears, and replacing them with positive belief statements. Remember, this is your baby's birth. You have the final say in who is there. This is your fundamental right.

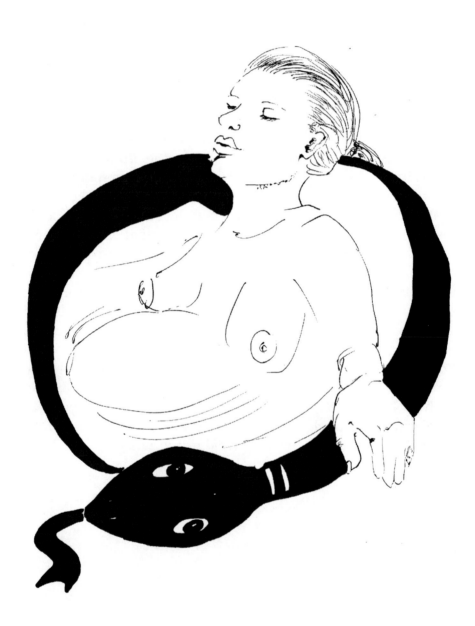

The Birth Fire

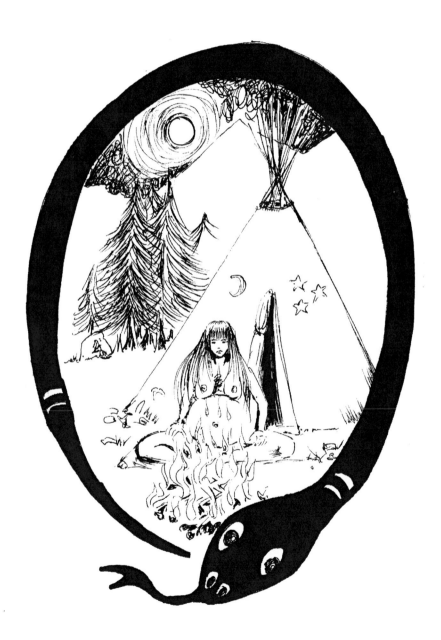

Heat and warmth have always been associated with childbirth. In modern times, most people only associate them with boiling water to sterilise things!

Building a fire for childbirth was done for practical purposes, as well as ceremonially. The warmth from the fire ensured comfort for the birthing mother, and supported her after birth when she was likely to become cold or exhausted. Our tribal sisters knew that keeping the mother warm with a fire helped her uterus to shrink back to pre-pregnancy size.

Our modern birthing practitioners could learn a lot from our tribal sisters. Thai women, for example, would make a bed of banana leaves for the mother to lie on. Her belly was kept as warm as possible. The use of fire as a post-partum support tended to last for at least seven days. During this time, the mother was regularly massaged with a sponge. She also had steam baths. Burmese and Vietnamese women also utilised steamy baths. The birth fire was integral to supporting a mother after birth in many places ~ including Borneo, Sumatra, the Philippines, Sarawak and Malaya. In New Guinea and the Solomon islands, a new mother has her abdomen wrapped in leaves which have been warmed. Throughout the Pacific islands, various fire treatments were used.

Further south, in Australia, the Tiwi create a fire during labour. After birth has occurred, the fire is put out, so the mother (who has birthed quietly in the bush) can squat over the warmed earth. Her tribal sisters will have wrapped some hot ash in cloth and placed it on her abdomen. It would seem a much gentler way than some of the fire treatments in other countries. The Hopi of North America used what was called a fire rest for their birthing women. They created a heated sand bed for the mother to lie on. She also had the benefit of rocks which had been heat treated. They were placed by her feet. A similar practice was very common in other North American tribes, where a pit was heated with fire, then lined with sand or ash, for the mother to lie in. Down south, in Guatemala and Mexico, the heat was used in a manner not dissimilar to the steam baths. They used grasses which had been wetted, to give the mother a sweat bath.

Indian women used warm baths straight after birth and throughout post partum. Some tribes in India, such as the Thakurs, would wrap heated cow dung or sand on the mother's belly. The idea was to induce perspiration, so she could release toxins. Hot baths were also used in west Africa.

Regardless of the tribe, the use of heat had four main purposes: to prevent excessive bleeding; to bring down the mother's milk; to offer her post-birth comfort; and to help shrink the uterus.

**Regardless of the tribe,
the use of heat
had four main purposes:
to prevent excessive bleeding;
to bring down the mother's milk;
to offer her post-birth comfort;
and to help shrink the uterus.**

The five needs of every baby

Our mother's heartbeat is the soundtrack to our life.

Just prior to birth, a baby's body produces adrenal hormones. Too much of these will bring on shock. Sustained adrenal hormone coursing through an infant's body will kill. It is absolutely crucial that we slow and stop these hormones by honouring the five post birth needs of every baby.

Vision

It is important for a baby to see a face at delivery. When it does so, the baby will smile within forty five minutes of birth. Otherwise it will take weeks or months. Most modern births lead to loss of awareness, which can take months for the baby to regain.

Hearing

Baby needs to hear his mother's voice, and her heart beat, immediately after birth. Most mothers instinctively put their baby to the left breast, which is where the heart is.

Colostrum

All the mother's immunities which she has received throughout her life are transferred to baby through colostrum, which also brings the baby's hormones into balance.

Colostrum is rich in Vitamin A, copper and zinc. This first liquid from a mother's breasts is so rich in antibodies that it is capable of protecting against measles, polio, mumps and other diseases, as well as infections of the chest, such as pneumonia and influenza.

It is every baby's birthright to receive colostrum. Unfortunately, many Western babies do not receive it, and sadly, there are tribal babies who also miss out on this important gift from Nature. Studies of adults with a history of violence, depression, suicidal tendencies and criminal acts show that they all have in common a reduced level of serotonin in their bodies. This is a chemical in the brain, the level of which, is reduced when the affectionate loving and bonding between mother and child aren't adequate. Colostrum contains tryptophan, an essential ingredient for developing serotonin. This isn't in artificial milk. And this is why we have such high rates of clinical depression.

Throughout our mammalian history we've had these two aspects ~ the physiological component of breastfeeding, and the psychological benefits of mother love and attention from continuous contact ~ supporting each other in order to help the babies of our species grow their brains and bodies optimally.

All the messages of well-being that a baby receives from his mother's continual heart to heart connections are relayed to the midbrain (the emotional centre/heart of the brain), and make his world stable. Nature assures us of his intelligence and social compatibility. Bonding holds life together.

Nature intends for us to bond with mother at birth. Historically, the violent cultures and tribes were those which withheld colostrum. This was done to make their people more aggressive and warrior-like. Violence breeds violence. When a baby's need for colostrum is not met, the results are with society for life.

Modern births are one of the greatest inhibitors to successful breastfeeding. Interference with our birthing hormones, physically or emotionally, can lead to many breastfeeding complications, such as plugged ducts, engorgement, abscesses, stress, and belief in Insufficient Milk Syndrome.

Insufficient Milk Syndrome is based on the idea that some women can't make milk. This is untrue. In fact, ISM only exists in places where it is easy access to artificial infant milk.

In tribal societies, we find that any woman can produce milk, and very often women beyond menopausal age are breastfeeding babies in the tribe. What's even more fascinating is that women who haven't had children are able to make milk as well. This is found in cultures around the world which haven't been force-fed the artificial milk concept.

Touch

Skin to skin contact is vital. All mammals lick or rub their newborns to stimulate the nerves in the skin. We mistakenly assume that they're just washing them clean! A baby needs its mother's skin, not a blanket, or weighing scales, or to be swaddled. The baby needs his mother's skin.

Smell

A newborn baby's highly sensitive sense of smell means he can pick out his mother from a room full of women.

Vision, hearing, colostrum, touch and smell. Five needs all met by the natural practice of breastfeeding, which is available to any woman with undamaged breasts, anywhere around the world.
The reinforcement of a mother's heartbeat after birth is absolutely VITAL to bonding. Bringing mother's and baby's hearts together again after birth allows emotional imprinting on the baby's midbrain. This MUST keep happening, to seal the bond. Birth is complete. This is what Nature planned. This is her blueprint.

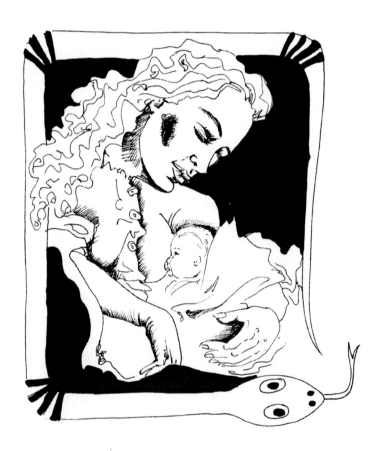

The Babymoon

A newborn baby is exquisitely sensitive to every sensation. Millions of years of human evolution have etched into every cell of his body the expectation that he will be held, will smell his mother, and will breastfeed at birth. If I could wave a wand and guide how babies are welcomed into our world, it would be something like this:

[] Include warm water: Either labour and birth in water, or introduce your baby to warm water immediately after birth, to reassure the baby as he leaves the warm world of amniotic fluid. Ensure the baby is warm enough and his body is covered.

[] Low lighting: Some people use dim lamps or several beeswax/plant-based candles to light the room. Be aware of the huge shock of emerging from the dark insides of a mother's belly into a brightly-lit room.

[] Lavender essential oil: Subtly scenting the room, lavender is calming and relaxing for all concerned, including babe.

[] Quiet: As with light, be aware of the huge transition from the inside world of utero, to our world, where the noise is no longer muffled. Be sensitive.

[] Gentle singing or humming: Especially if the mother has been singing throughout pregnancy, this will help to welcome the baby.

[] Softly spoken words of welcome: Parents can use this time to verbalise their love, by speaking softly to their new baby.

[] Breastfeed: Do this as soon as possible after birth. If baby doesn't immediately appear interested in feeding, ensure he is held in his mother's arms, next to her heartbeat. This is vital for bonding.

[] Consider a lotus birth: At the very least, delay cutting the cord for an hour or two. Cord blood belongs to the baby. Allow time for the transfusion, physical and psychic, to occur.

[] Engage in a Babymoon: Keep visitors to a minimum for a few weeks. Honour this transition time for all of you, and especially for the baby. Let your baby get used to his new home and way of living.

Man-made law

Planned unassisted childbirth is legal in the UK. Unfortunately, it's not a commonly-known law, hence the difficulty some families have come across when registering their baby's birth. The law states that the mother must not be attended in labour by someone not registered as a midwife or doctor. The mother always has the right to birth her own baby without assistance or supervision. A baby's father can legally be present at an unassisted birth. There is often confusion by people who don't understand the law and believe it means that he can't support his partner while she gives birth.

Some countries in Europe are not keen to acknowledge unassisted childbirth. Regardless of which country you're in, it's always best to wait several weeks before registering the child's birth. When affirming your easy birth, you should also see yourself, your partner and your baby as being safe afterwards.

The UK's Department of Health states "There are risks involved and we do not recommend freebirth". There are risks in every aspect of life. I risk my life every time I walk down my stairs, or plug in an electrical appliance, or put food in my mouth or cross the road. The DoH doesn't issue statements telling us that to 'live' is dangerous. To use a government body as the authoritative voice of childbirth is ludicrous. The only true expert of birth is an intuitive woman in labour. No birth professional, such as an obstetrician, is going to recommend freebirth/unassisted birth, simply because they're used to seeing what 'bad' births look like ~ and because autonomous birth doesn't earn them any money.

The official stance from The Royal College of Obstetricians and Gynaecologists (RCOG) is that they are "aware of the small number of women choosing unassisted childbirth. Whilst the RCOG fully supports normal birth and believes that every woman should have the right to give birth in an environment in which she feels comfortable, the safety and well-being of the mother and baby are paramount. Before choosing a place of birth, all women should be fully informed of the potential risks, which may include the need for intervention, transfer to hospital and/or pain relief. Obstetricians and midwives are concerned with the safety of both patients, mother and child." (Author's note: interesting that they use the word 'patient', as if to denote there is an illness or disease to be dealt with).

"The RCOG would like to stress that at present, the practice of freebirth is new to the UK and little research exists regarding its safety and success". Freebirth might be 'new' to the UK, but humanity has been practising birth like this since the dawn of civilisation.

Bear in mind that we're physiologically designed to catch our own baby at birth. A woman always has the ability to draw on Human Rights law, even if her own country isn't accommodating of planned unassisted birth.

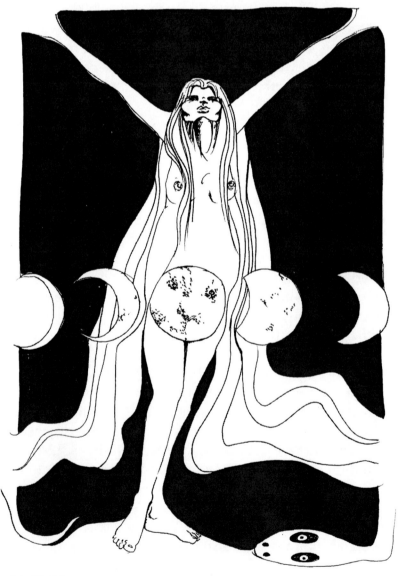

The mother
always has the right
to birth her own baby
without
assistance
or
supervision.

Universal Law

Man-made law is based on fear and control. Universal Law is based on love, and the power of attraction. The latter recognises us as multi-dimensional beings, with physical, emotional, mental, astral and etheric bodies. Man-made law only sees the visible side of us.

As birthing women, we have a choice, to step into fear or into love. Regardless of the laws created by man to protect women and babies in birth, it's clear to see that true protection is not about disempowering women. Any law which instructs a woman on where, when and how to give birth is *not* protecting her, but causing her to relinquish her own power and birthing majesty. We have a choice: to birth inside the obstetrical box, or to leave it behind and birth wherever and however we want; free to welcome our babies in a space and place of love and gratitude.

The future of unassisted birth

Humans are the only mammals which socialise at birth. I believe more and more women are waking up to the power within them, and also realising that birth is sacred, beautiful and of Divine origin. In doing so, they are questioning the dominant birth culture, which hypnotises us into believing the exact opposite. The more often that Birthkeepers can tell their stories, the sooner we'll reach the 'tipping point' ~ that moment when things become the norm in our culture. It begins invisibly, and then is made visible.

And so it is with unassisted birth. We enter the journey in a way that leaves us invisible to the culture, and then we re-enter, babe in arms, to tell our stories.

What can we learn from our ancestresses?

Attitudes to birth must be positive if we wish to see women birth with ease. Our culture has us believing birth to be dangerous and deadly, and so we see ourselves as victims and yield ourselves ~ body and soul ~ to the medical profession in order that we'll be saved. Tribal women knew the power of birth was with them, and not with someone or something outside of themselves.

Our ancestresses also showed us the importance of not having strangers at our birthing. By all means have an attendant, but ensure it is someone you feel love for. Familiarity in birth is everything. It is certainly not the time to be meeting your midwife or trainee midwives or obstetricians. Nor is it the time to leave your nest and drive to a hospital.

Someone in your lifetime will know women who've had difficult births, and then cite this as a reason for needing medical care at birth. However, if we look beyond the fear veneer, we see that our elderly women did not have lifestyles conducive to good health. Many had vitamin and mineral deficiencies, others had sexual diseases, didn't exercise adequately or receive proper amounts of sunlight on their skin.

You might argue that women of our modern birthing age are not necessarily likely to suffer from such things. Although our diets in general are better, many of us are nutrient deficient, too. The most fundamental thing to remember though, is that we have inherited the fears of our grandmothers: their pain and deaths connected with childbirth are the messages we receive. Sadly, we receive them without understanding that we take on these belief systems as our own, and then pass them on to our daughters, sisters and nieces. And so the cycle of fear continues.

In order to birth easily, effortlessly and beautifully, we must release all fears ~ both our own, and our grandmothers'.

The key to all aspects of our life is to rediscover the magic of simple living, for it is here we find both our questions and answers. By doing so, we remember within every cell of our being that humans have been birthed vaginally without major incident for millions of years.

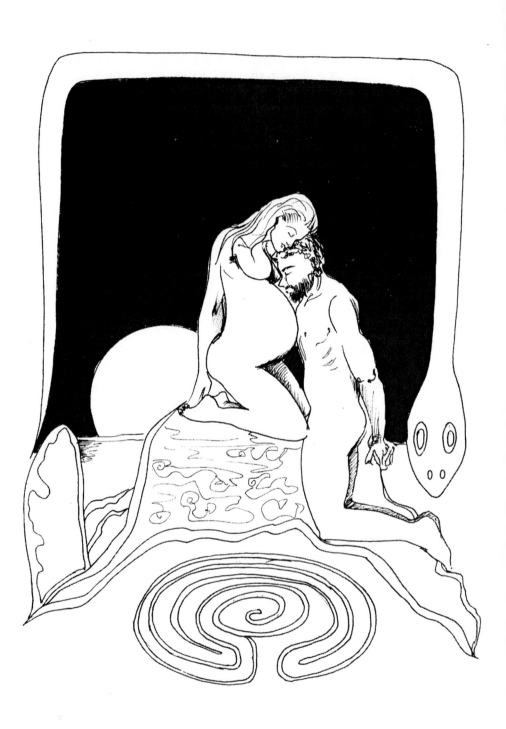

The Birthkeepers Speak

Reading other women's birth stories transports us to an area not visited in everyday life. We can learn so much from others' experiences, though we never truly understand birth until we walk through those doors ourselves.

It is vital to seek out positive, inspiring birth stories: to read of the journeys where women took control of their birthing story, and brought it alive with their consciousness.

Regardless of the birth place and birth plan you have, take heart and wisdom from the stories which follow, for they tell us how magical birth can be when left free of medical intervention.

Jack's unassisted birth
written by Amelia Curtis

We are threatened in the ultimate way: by the fear of death ~ death of our new baby, ourselves, or worse still, both.

I needed to face the possibility of death; and the truth that some women and babies do die in the birthing process ~ naturally, as well as within 'medically protected' ones.

And the truth is also that many of us die just living our lives. And of course, the truth is: we die...

Not that I realised it at the time, but Jack's unassisted childbirth was a real ~ as in not conceptual ~ initiation rite into gaining my full power as a living, breathing, passionate and sacred, natural woman and mother.

Every woman has the potential to become like this, and every man has the power and potential to become a living, breathing, passionate protector of this Divine femininity.

Conventional medical childbirth is about the need to control females. Men and women are in such a state of degeneration that their consciousness has no ability to trust Nature, and certainly no ability to trust women's intuition in the birthing process.

My own intuition towards birthing unassisted came about after I changed my diet to a more natural one. I read a book which included the story about the author's unassisted childbirth, and it was immediately apparent to me that this was how I would birth my next child.

I had already given birth to my firstborn, Lily; and at the time I had this birthing revelation and insight, she was about one and a half. Her birth hadn't gone to plan. I was only 22, and although I was a somewhat feisty character, I still felt dominated by those seen to be in positions of authority. Being emotionally immature, what I needed was a protective connection to some powerful, intuitive females. Due to the culture we are brought (or is that dragged, barbarically?) up in, I knew no-one I could trust on this level, and although I had wanted a natural birth, I was swayed by the fearful, medical midwives and doctors into being artificially induced after being 14 days 'overdue'. I vividly remember the process, and my heart ached and cried to be respected properly.

Initially, 'to get me started', I was, what can only be described in my mind, as 'attacked' by one of the midwives at the hospital. I realise what she did was normal procedure, but her lack of respect and emotion about what was happening was a gross misunderstanding of the beauty and awesomeness of the birthing process, and the female form. She stuck and pushed, with no lubrication on her rubber gloves, two fingers inside my vagina, and swept a pessary hard into my cervix. I remember the intense feeling of humiliation and shock as this happened, and moved my body back against the bed I was lying on, only to be told in an authoritative and cold voice to keep still. I also remember the relief at being told that this midwife was soon to go off duty, and that another midwife would replace her.

When I met the next midwife, although she seemed nicer than the last, she was still obviously indoctrinated against the natural birthing process, as she decided to induce me further, by breaking my waters. Just stepping into a hospital environment was, at the time, enough to take away what little feminine power I had, and I found it almost impossible to say "no". I also had no real emotional understanding of what was about to happen.

With what looked like a crochet hook, the midwife stuck this instrument into my vagina and tore the baby's protective bag, until water started to run out of me. Almost instantly, I went into full-blown labour, and started having contractions every few minutes that were very painful and long. They forced me into a state of panic, as I had none of the build-up that my mind had prepared me for. I had been led to believe that within the birthing process the body naturally starts opening the cervix slowly, and builds up in intensity as the baby nears birth; and here I was hanging over the bed as soon as labour began, in complete agony every few minutes. I reached unashamedly for the gas and air, and focused with all of my might on getting through each contraction, even though I was completely spaced-out and didn't really know where I was, or what I was doing. The midwife somehow managed to get me into a warm bath to help me to cope, and I spent two hours in there before the pain became so unbearable that I started asking for an epidural ~ something I hadn't even considered being an option before I was artificially induced.

Little did I know, also having been led to believe that the birthing process is a lot longer than a few hours, that I was in transition, and I would soon be meeting my daughter. I remember not knowing what was going on other than needing serious relief from the pain. As I got onto the bed to get ready for my epidural, the midwife asked me if I needed to push. I didn't actually know, my mind being so disorientated, and I certainly did not have any desire to push; but I gave it a try anyway, and actually felt some immediate relief from the pain.

By the time the epidural anaesthetist entered the room, my baby was half way out, and with some intense effort on my part (that, in hindsight after Jack's birth, can only be described as being as artificial as the 'crochet' needle and pessary), I pushed Lily out within eleven minutes. More medical procedures followed that were, in their own way, designed to 'help', but of course, these were as traumatic as the labour, and I went home with my baby, dis-empowered and shocked.

I have told this story to give some context to why my unassisted childbirth was such a deep and profound initiation rite, and also as a way to connect with those who have been through similar experiences.

When I found out I was pregnant with my son, Jack, I decided not only was I going to try for an unassisted birth, but that, as much as possible, I would avoid the medical procedures in pregnancy, also. Being 25, I was still not emotionally mature or in my full power, and decided that I had best get some medical care when I reached six months of my pregnancy (now I would not bother with any of it). It was not the medical care I was really after, but peace of mind that I wasn't challenging the status-quo too much, and drawing to me unwanted attention.

The midwife I was assigned was the most senior one. It would probably be an understatement to say she found my character somewhat challenging. Firstly, she was shocked I had left it so long to see someone in authority, and then horrified that I was refusing to have an ultrascan. She said she had never had any woman refuse a scan, and was very unhappy that she would not know that everything was as it should be before the birth. I did not fill her in on my planned unassisted birth, letting her believe I intended on having a natural birth at home, with a midwife present. Interestingly, I was never actually asked if I wanted a midwife present, it was just presumed I would ~ a bit like scientists presuming humans are currently at the pinnacle of evolution, even though we have created a level of destruction that has forced us to crisis point on many levels of our interaction with each other and the Earth we live upon.

I did not feel in any way safe with this midwife, and even though there is no law against unassisted birth in the UK, this was a sacred decision, and I was keeping it a secret.

At around seven months, she got me to see a doctor, as she was apparently worried that there was not enough fluid in the baby's sac, and that the baby's kidneys were possibly failing. They both convinced me to have an emergency ultrascan the next day, and I went home feeling scared and alone. The father of the baby, who was my partner at the time, and who had been supporting me throughout my pregnancy, was in Spain, and I hadn't bonded with any of the local women. The only place to go was inward, and I decided that before I went to the ultrascan in the morning, I would have a deep meditation with my baby.

As I dropped myself down into a deep state of consciousness, I found an energetic space with my baby, where it became apparent that he (I knew it was a boy) was completely well and healthy, and there was absolutely no need for me to blast his brain with radiation in order to tell me this truth! Feeling stronger and confident, I did not turn up to my appointment the next morning, and I reckon the midwife must have drunk a stiff whisky that evening after I had told her that I'd meditated with the baby, and there'd been no need to go for the emergency scan. Outside of this medical part of my pregnancy, the spiritual aspect, and feeling of initiation, were dominated by something that could be seen as more powerful: my own doubting and fearful mind. I can not really describe how overwhelming at times this voice was. We are told throughout our lives (subliminally and blatantly), as women, not only can we not trust ourselves, full stop, and need to hand over our power to men, or those seen in a position of knowledge and authority, but as birthing women we really need to be protected by those who have been fully-trained medically. There would appear to be no messages that the birthing process is actually natural, and that a woman's body knows how to give birth, just like any other species that gives birth on the planet.

We are threatened in the ultimate way: by the fear of death ~ death of our new baby, ourselves, or worse still, both. And this is what I needed to face in order to take full responsibility for the birth of my baby, and ultimately, the birth of my true, authentic, internally-directed, Divine and natural self. I needed to face the possibility of death; and the truth that some women and babies do die in the birthing process ~ naturally, as well as within 'medically protected' ones. And the truth is also that many of us die just living our lives. And of course, the truth is: we die. If I couldn't face this truth, then I would be forever bound to handing over my power to anyone who offered me some suggested protection from this truth. By the time the birth of Jack came around, I had faced many of my deepest fears through the use of deep meditation and months of gentle re-birthing. I was still a little frightened of the unknown, but I had a deep sense that the birth would be incredible, and life-changing. I was going overdue, and thankfully, my midwife was on holiday when I needed to deal with the whole issue of being artificially-induced again. I told the midwife who was on-call that I was willing to wait a few weeks before this needed to be discussed in any seriousness; and on the 10th day after the 'due date', I went into labour.

I had been affirming throughout my pregnancy the intention of having a pain-free birth, and on good days I would even affirm an orgasmic childbirth. In the afternoon, I'd had the first sign that something was happening, when I had a sensation of a knot untying in my cervix. I'm not quite sure what it was, and did not even realise it was significant at the time, but remember thinking it was an unusual sensation. About five hours later, the first real signs of labour occurred, and I had a pain-free sensation ride through my cervix, gently, for about 15 seconds, at intervals of about 10 minutes. Although they were not painful, I would stand facing the wall with my hands pushing against it in front of me, whilst I moved my legs in a walking manner, breathing deeply. My partner phoned a friend of mine to help him get everything ready, and my daughter's paternal grandma was there, helping with Lily, and washing up. I was already starting to slip into a sensitive and energetic space, and I remember the feeling of really needing the right people around after Lily's grandma entered my personal space to ask if my waters had broken yet. I could feel her fear, and although it had been discussed beforehand that she may be present for the birth, I knew in that moment that there was no way she could be. I did not have the courage at the time to ask her to leave, but she must have picked up on the vibe, because not long after, she decided to go home to get some sleep. I was very relieved when she left, and felt myself relax into the process that was unfolding. Lily was now in bed, and the birthing pool was ready for me to enter. I remember feeling completely protected and enveloped, within the water. Candles were lit, and relaxing music was playing softly in the background; the energy and ambience was obviously completely different than that of my first birth, and I felt deliciously content with how things were going.

The contractions were still not in any way painful, and I seemed to be slipping into a deeply altered state of consciousness. I was having intense energetic eye connection with the father of my son, and was seeing bright colours of energy swirling around his head. I went into a spontaneous chant, and although I practised spiritual and shamanic techniques at the time, chanting had never been something that particularly interested me. I can't remember what sounds I was chanting, but I remember them completely grounding my mind. My body went into spontaneous movement that mimicked Tai Chi, and was completely synchronised: flowing and opening as if some part of my deeper self was taking over.

Even though during my pregnancy I had been affirming having a pain-free birth, I was still shocked at how pain-free it was! It is difficult for me to describe the sensations, but I can only say that I could feel a sensation of opening in my cervix, or something happening in my vagina, but it just was not painful in any way. I rested in this state of consciousness for possibly a few hours, although time had become irrelevant: and then my daughter awoke.

The first thought that crossed my mind when this happened was a fearful one, as I wondered how Lily might cope watching me give birth. This thought, due to the shift in my conscious orientation, was enough to make the next contraction painful, and I remember my body pulling me up out of the cross-legged meditative position I'd been in, to a more primal one where I was on my knees, with my arms and head leaning against the side of the pool. From that moment every contraction was painful, and I remember thinking how shockingly connected pain/pleasure is to our state of mind. After perhaps 15 minutes of contractions that were getting closer together and more painful in their nature, I slipped into a completely different state of consciousness to the past few hours.

I really wanted to get out of the birthing pool, and yet because I knew that my friend and partner were into waterbirths, I felt uncomfortable owning this bodily need. As stupid as it sounds now, I became dominated by thoughts about what I believed my friend, and partner, would want me to do, even though I know, in hindsight, that both would have wanted me to do exactly what I needed to! In fact, I remember them asking me, as they saw my mind flip into panic, what I wanted to do, and although my body wanted desperately to get out of the pool, my mind, out of its deluded desire to please my friend and my partner, stayed in. It sounds so ludicrous to me now, and I can see clearly it was only my pattern of seeking approval from others rearing its head again.

The birthing process reflects who we are at the time. Although I was taking my power back by birthing medically-unassisted, I obviously had some work to do in fully owning my truth. My mind kept me under rigid control for about half an hour, not being able to own my body's desire until it reached a critical point, and my body almost threw me out of the birthing pool. Again, as in the birth of my first child, I hadn't realised I had slipped into transition, and I remember feeling I was losing my mind and not really knowing what was going on.

Although I was conscious, I was also in a state of dis-orientation, and I walked up and down the stairs a few times, making loud primal noises whilst bearing down, intuitively and naturally, when I reached a contraction. After doing this for about 15 minutes, and feeling the force of gravity had done what it needed to do, I felt sure that the baby was about to arrive; and without any pressure from either my own mind, or that of my friend or partner, I wanted to get back in the pool to give birth.

After getting back into the pool, which had been topped up with warm water to make it the right temperature, I adopted a natural position that felt right to give birth in. I had about another 15 contractions; all, I have to admit, were incredibly intense, and I had to focus my mind to get through each one. Then, almost out of nowhere, I felt this intense wave of energy course through my body, directing me into an even more aligned position ready for the baby to come out. I had already come across much literature about not pushing the baby out, and knew this was something I wanted to practise, but had no real idea what that really meant in terms of the baby being released through the birthing canal and into my arms. This part of the birth with Jack blows my mind to this day, as my body completely took over from my mind. The first body-directed push waved over me, and the waters broke, and Jack's head crowned. I put my hand down to touch his head, shouting that the baby was coming. The second body-directed push that waved through me, brought out the head, and the third brought out the rest of his body.

I couldn't believe how quickly this part had all happened, and how naturally. I scooped up my baby, and as he came out of the water he was actually asleep! He lay on my chest for a while, and I remember thinking how pink, healthy, calm, and content he looked. After a while he opened his eyes, and started to breastfeed. I slowly got out of the pool and carried him over to the sofa, where I was wrapped lovingly in a warm towel.

Within minutes of giving birth, the placenta delivered in just one contraction. I lay it on another towel, and cleared up the small amount of blood. Jack and I rested peacefully for about 45 minutes, before we called a midwife to come around and check everything was ok.

I admit I was not completely honest with the midwife about what had happened, and if the truth be known, even though I think she knew this, she did seem very respectful of me and the baby, so that I suspected she might have been the kind of midwife who would have been in awe of what I did. Something interesting that she commented on was that she had never seen such a thick bag before; I had eaten a nutritionally-dense diet throughout most of my pregnancy, and especially in the last three months. Considering the bag protects the baby from resting on its own cord and restricting oxygen supply, I have pondered whether it is crucially important for this to stay intact until the baby is literally about to come out of the birthing canal. Would diet have any influence over how strong a bag is, and therefore possibly dictate when the waters break? Could it be an important part of the birthing process for this to stay intact until the very end? What does this mean in terms of having the waters artificially broken before the baby is ready to come down the birthing canal?

When Veronika first asked me to write my story for this book, I felt a strong desire to do it. A while ago, after my unassisted birth and the changes it brought about to my character and life, I had considered starting up an organisation in the UK on unassisted birth. So writing my story to help inspire others, and bring a correction in alignment to the truth that we are living, breathing, passionate, natural, sacred women that can be trusted to give birth to our own babies ~ all of us ~ brings me joy.

How women are treated, and in particular, mothers, is a reflection of our culture and tribal consciousness. It would appear right now, for various reasons (that are too lengthy to explore here), that we are living within a culture of such pervasive misogyny that it has blinded the eyes of many women and men against the truth of what it means to be a birthing woman in today's culture. The practices that are all too routine, are so traumatic for mothers and babies, that the scars can last a lifetime.

All birthing mothers need to be completely respected and energetically held in love and trust. Ultimately, our bodies know how to give birth, and it can surely only be a sign of insanity that we would ever trust anything else.

It took me many months to be able to write this. And although at one time in my life I was always able to write easily and effortlessly, on demand, changes in my consciousness over the last few years have put me in touch with such powerful and multi-layered truths, that I now find it more difficult to coherently express myself in a way that I feel will be understood. Ironically, I need to wait patiently for the words to come to me in a stream that dictates their expression. I was getting very 'overdue' with writing these words for Veronika, and yet I couldn't buckle to any internal pressure (it would have only blocked the process more, anyway), and I chose to trust that if my story was to be included in the book, I was going to write it at just the right time.

Just like a mental pregnancy, I could feel these words brewing in my mind, creating themselves, whilst giving me some more life experiences that were needed before they could come into full expression. At the same time, I was going through, at 32, another initiation rite that had exactly the same theme running through it. That is, to fully claim my power as a woman and mother, as the feminine expression of creation.

After having come through a recent deep level of healing, I felt the words for this article were ready to appear. I wrote to Veronika to ask if I was too late, and her response was that only the day before had she crossed me of her list of contributors, as she was ready to put the whole book together. Needless to say the timing was impeccable, and the article appeared within a few days, ready for the book to be put together. Of course, I understood Veronika's need to take me off the list. In the world of material creation it's important for harmonious flow to have deadlines that are met. I knew she had really waited long enough, and she also knew I had been going through some powerful life changes that were all-consuming.

The birth process is completely different from that of creating a book. Birthing mothers and their babies are living, breathing, Divine creations, going through the most powerful, intense and real-life transition they will ever go through. To not have this respected by the medical birthing world is a tragedy that is so deeply traumatic, that it is too painful for many to fully own. I believe it is up to each individual to fully gain their power again. For us women, it is to truly feel our Divine awesomeness, and to trust our bodies and our intuition within the birthing process.

For some of us, we are choosing to birth unassisted, and for other women it means surrounding themselves with respectful, intuitive women whilst birthing; and thankfully there are some conscious midwives. I've met some on my journey since having Jack. But truthfully, there are not enough, and I sense that more and more women will be taking (or at least seriously considering taking) their full power back in the birthing process by choosing to birth completely unassisted, as Nature intended. If you're such a woman, I encourage you to trust yourself, and to trust the Divine intelligence that penetrates every living cell in your body. Your body truly knows how to give birth.

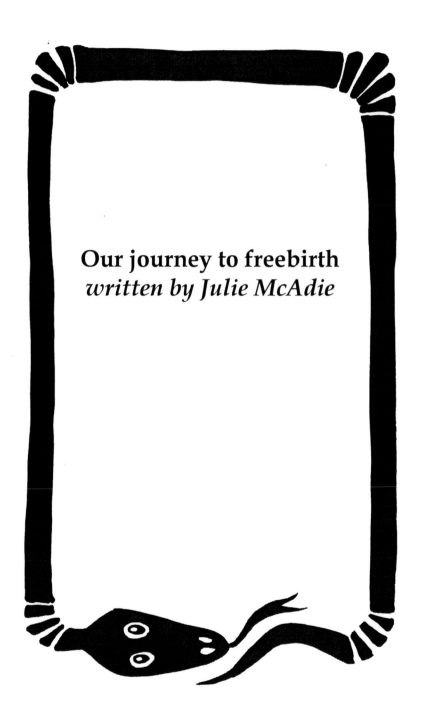

Our journey to freebirth
written by Julie McAdie

My first son, Callum, had been born in hospital ~ an experience which had seriously traumatised me. His was a 'natural' birth, lasting six hours, and without pain relief (of which I am very proud).

However, throughout his birth I was manipulated and subtly threatened by the midwives, who felt things were taking too long; I was strapped to a monitor the whole time; unnecessary episiotomy; filthy hospital, etc. This time things would be so different. I was in charge!

Our journey to freebirth began one afternoon as I was sitting face to face with a community midwife in my local doctor's surgery ~ a look of horror on her face. I was about 12 weeks pregnant with my second child, my first child with my husband, Dan. On asking me which hospital I would like to give birth in, I announced that I wanted to have my baby at home. She did not react the way I had anticipated! She was mortified, and proceeded to tell me how busy the community midwife team was, and chances were that there wouldn't be two midwives available on the day I went into labour, so I would have to "sign something" to say that I accepted this possibility, and would go to the hospital if that occurred. Our nearest hospital delivers thousands of babies a year, like a baby factory, and had recently been in the news, and put on emergency measures by the National Health Service (NHS), because a high number of mothers had, sadly, died there. This midwife was not kind, caring or at all interested in my wishes. She tried to make me feel selfish and irresponsible; I felt shocked and bullied.

I endured a few more appointments with this midwife before making various complaints. I felt very stressed during this period, and worried that I would be forced to have the kind of birth my instincts did not want. I so desperately wanted to have a homebirth. I was assigned a new NHS midwife, who would come to my home to carry out my appointments. Penny was lovely, a midwife committed to seeing through to the birth and beyond, with every mother she was assigned. I would have continuity in my care.

However, the seed of freebirth had already been planted in my mind. All the trouble with the original midwife had forced me to look into other options. Hiring a private midwife was beyond our means. We visited a Birth Centre, described as a 'home from home' ~ the sterile corridors, hospital beds and sheets did not much resemble my home! So I read books such as Unassisted Birth by Laura Kaplan Shanley, The Power Of Pleasurable Childbirth by Laurie A. Morgan, and Ina May Gaskin's Spiritual Midwifery. I searched for forums and articles on the internet. There was little UK based information, but I knew I couldn't be the only woman in the country thinking about unassisted birth. It was such a joy to discover that freebirthing was a possibility, that there were many women around the world who had already done it.

I continued my appointments with Penny; I enjoyed her reassurance, and confidence in homebirth.

But I didn't tell her of my ultimate plan to freebirth, as I wasn't sure of the legal issues surrounding it; and I did not want her to be concerned for me.

I discussed birthing unassisted with my husband. He had been reluctant about even homebirthing at first, but slowly he came around to the idea of delivering our baby, just the two of us. I showed him various freebirth stories and sections of books, which he would read at first, but after a while he stopped showing an interest. This worried me at the time, and I thought perhaps he didn't really believe I would go through with it, and would want to call the midwife when labour started. I now realise that he had developed his own inner strength around the issue, and was self-confident enough to go ahead without reading any more information.

Dan's support was essential to me. I knew in my heart that I could not have strangers in my space when giving birth. I didn't want a stranger touching me or putting a hand inside me to check dilation. Only my husband is permitted that intimacy with me. I knew that any midwife would need to check things, make suggestions, try to orchestrate my baby's birth ~ that is what they are trained to do. I simply could not tolerate that intrusion.

My first son, Callum, had been born in hospital ~ an experience which had seriously traumatised me. His was a 'natural' birth, lasting six hours, and without pain relief (of which I am very proud). However, throughout his birth I was manipulated and subtly threatened by the midwives, who felt things were taking too long; I was strapped to a monitor the whole time; unnecessary episiotomy; filthy hospital, etc. This time things would be so different. I was in charge!

Throughout my second pregnancy I went through stages of questioning and doubting my decision ~ with periods of isolation because I knew no-one else who was planning to freebirth. I told only a few of my friends what we had planned, as I realised most people would not understand at all and might be afraid for me (and my sanity), and perhaps make me afraid in the process. One well-meaning friend offered me a lift to the hospital whenever I needed it, day or night. I had no intention of taking her up on it.

I practised the art of positive thinking. I imagined the birth going beautifully, just as I wanted it to: visualising how it would all unfold.

We purchased a lovely birth pool, and had fun setting it up in the kitchen, checking for any leaks and having a little swim! I chose relaxing music cds I might want to listen to in labour. I knew I would have a short labour, and that the baby would arrive quickly.

I had hoped that Callum would like to witness his sister being born, but he was adamant he didn't wish to be there, and I didn't push him. This prompted some discussion about where Callum could go during the birth. I concluded, however, that it wouldn't be a proper homebirth if one family member had to leave the home for the birth to take place! I had a strong intuition that the birth would happen at night, and Callum would sleep peacefully through the entire event, so I trusted that. I was so looking forward to meeting my baby girl that I became a little despondent when my due date came and went. I knew that she would come only when she was absolutely ready, but I was big and heavy, and every day that I was overdue felt like a week.

At about 7.30pm on Friday the 9th of November 2007, nine days after she was due, my waters broke, and the most exciting phase of our freebirth journey began. I was standing on a towel by the kitchen sink, desperately trying to finish the washing up whilst my waters gushed out. I was adamant I would not be giving birth next to dirty dishes! Dan quickly leapt into action, moving table and chairs out of the kitchen, and setting up the birth pool. We didn't hang around; we knew things would progress quickly. So I finished up my chores and put Callum to bed. Bless him, he watched Dan setting up the birth pool but didn't catch on that this meant our baby was coming. I didn't say anything, but smiled to myself in anticipation of surprising him with his new sister in the morning.

When I returned to the kitchen, my wonderful husband had set everything up beautifully. The windows were covered with makeshift blinds (we are in a ground floor flat, and didn't want the neighbours peeking in); he had set tea lights burning in their holders, and the birth pool was filled to the perfect depth and temperature; towels were to hand, and he had set a chair for himself next to the pool. I had prepared a box full of things I thought I might need: various Bach Flower Remedies; snack bars; more candles; soothing music cds; mineral water; a quartz crystal I had been given to put in the pool water; a flannel; lavender oil, that sort of thing.

We decided to set up the laptop computer in the kitchen, and watch one of our favourite films, Amelie, to pass some time.

My contractions had begun; they were gentle, and I soon got into a rhythm with them. I got straight into the pool and enjoyed the warmth and support the water offered me. I was very aware that had a midwife been present she would have discouraged me from getting in so early on, so I felt pleased that I was free to go with my intuition. I loved the freedom I had to move into whatever position felt comfortable. As the contractions progressed, I favoured being on all fours, rocking my hips from side to side, or kneeling up, holding onto the pool's edge. I watched bits of the film, but lost interest as my birthing picked up, and I drifted in my own little world.

I had been determined to have a fear-free birth, as I do believe (as Grantly Dick-Read details in his book, Childbirth Without Fear) that fear causes tension in the body; the tension causes pain, which in turn provokes more fear, and so the cycle continues. I kept affirming to myself "I am not afraid", "There is nothing to fear", "I can do this".

After an hour or so (we weren't really timing anything), my contractions moved down into a deeper level and I knew baby would be with us soon. I began to make low moaning sounds, much like a bellowing cow. These moans were completely involuntary, coming from somewhere deep within me. With each contraction, my husband pushed down on the base of my spine, and rubbed firmly in a circular motion to ease my discomfort. I had started to feel some pain, and with that I began to worry a bit; part of me thinking maybe we should call the midwife after all, but the contractions were always manageable, and I never felt overwhelmed. Dan encouraged me to relax. I had nothing to worry about.

Our baby's head started to crown, and I reached down to feel the very top of her head poking out. It then felt like nothing happened or moved for quite a long time, and I did worry that maybe something was wrong, and she was stuck.

I must have been in a strange head space, as I began to think maybe this was something other than the baby coming out of my body (I don't know what I thought it could have been!). I kept asking my husband "Are you sure it's the head?"

I shifted position at this point, my intuition telling me to stand up in the pool. Baby's head began to crown properly, then: and I made lots of loud bellowing sounds. I must add that up until this point I did not push at all, baby came down on her own, my body didn't need extra forced effort from me. However, as her head was coming and I was worrying a bit that it wasn't coming quickly enough, I did push just a little. I later regretted not trusting my body all the way, as I tore slightly. With Dan behind me, I leaned on the edge of the pool as my baby's head emerged. Apparently, she spat out some fluid, then her body slid out into my husband's hands. She cried a little after about five seconds. I turned around, stepped over her umbilical cord, sat back down in the water, and took our beautiful daughter in my arms. She was covered in a thick, white vernix. Her skin, at first, had a slightly purplish tint, but soon turned a beautiful pink. She was a lovely size. I was in a state of awe as I held my perfect little girl in my arms. I felt relief that she had arrived safely and appeared healthy and strong. I was so proud of my husband and myself for achieving our freebirth with strength and courage. The time was 10.25 pm, and labour had taken around three hours in total, just as I had known it would.

After half an hour of admiring our new addition, I began to feel cold, shaky and a little unwell. The placenta had not yet emerged, and baby's umbilical cord was quite short, so I was feeling uncomfortable. It was at this point that I decided I wanted Penny, the midwife, to come. I needed a fellow woman to be with me, to help me, and Penny was the only person we could call. Dan had not yet met Penny, and was a little reluctant to invite anyone into the private space we had created, but I needed her then, needed a woman's presence. So Dan went to call her. She must have thought she misheard him when he told her the baby had arrived, because I heard him say "No, the baby is already here". Apparently she was a bit cross with him on the phone, but she arrived at our home 15 minutes later, and didn't say a single negative word to us. At this stage the umbilical cord had stopped pulsating. Dan cut it and then had his first opportunity to properly hold his new daughter.

Penny encouraged me to step out of the birth pool, and this movement enabled the placenta to slip out. It was intact and healthy-looking. I was keen to examine it, having not had the chance to view my son's placenta five years previously. Penny helped to clean the baby and I up, and I got into bed for more cuddles with my newborn. Our baby was perfectly healthy, weighing a robust 9lbs. It felt so wonderful to be in my own comfortable bed in familiar surroundings. I was so thankful we had bypassed the unfamiliar, sterile hospital environment.

I think the midwife caught onto the fact that we had deliberately birthed without her, but we remained a little cagey about it. I know she felt disappointed at missing the event, as she genuinely enjoys helping women to birth at home. However, she was lovely to us throughout, and I will always remember her kindness.

After the birth, I recovered fairly quickly, and my small tears healed easily. A week later we chose the names Isobel Alice for our beautiful girl ~ Alice, after my great-grandmother, who had been born on the same date. Isobel has always been a very calm and contented baby, sleeping through the night from about a month onwards. I know this is down to her gentle introduction to the world. She's alert and wise, and has fitted perfectly into our family. She's adored by all of us.

I already look forward to experiencing another freebirth, should we be blessed in the future with another child. Next time, I would go the whole way with freebirth, having minimal or no contact with the NHS.

I cannot express enough just how proud I am of us and our freebirth. It was all so natural and empowering, free of fear and full of love, just as birth should be. The experience has changed my life. I am so much more confident and self assured now. It has bonded my husband and I even closer together, and I know we will remember Isobel's birth with joy, for the rest of our lives.

(Since writing this birth story, Julie has had another freebirth.)

*I had been determined
to have a fear-free birth, as I do believe
that fear causes tension in the body;
the tension causes pain,
which in turn provokes more fear,
and so the cycle continues.*

*I kept affirming to myself "I am not afraid",
"There is nothing to fear",
"I can do this".*

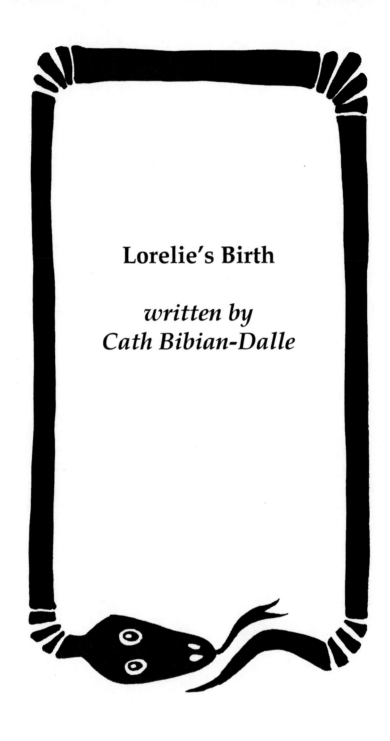

Lorelie's Birth

written by
Cath Bibian-Dalle

Like the peace following a huge storm,
at that time I knew I was in transition.
I just had to fully enjoy that peaceful moment
before finally having the chance
to meet our baby.

I am the third daughter out of four, born by planned caesarean section in 1973. Mum had been told her cervix was 'failing'. What a terrible word, what a dreadful expression.

Elena, my first daughter, was born, naturally, after a 38 hour labour, a transfer to hospital, induction, threats to have caesarean section, constant monitoring, etc. Not ideal, not peaceful, but so rewarding and empowering.

Tahlia, our second daughter, was born at home after a seven hour labour. We had an independent midwife who completely respected our will to let things progress and unfold at their own rhythm. She also supported us in times of doubt: such a wonderful experience, such an amazing lotus birthed baby who has grown into a happy-smiley-always-laughing toddler.

We became pregnant again in June 2007. My third baby, the same position in the family as me. What an amazing pregnancy. I was so connected with my baby, discovering prenatal communication, and enjoying relaxation sessions, meditation and talking to my baby. I felt so confident in this pregnancy, so strong, so blooming in all senses of the word. I felt I was completely trusting Nature, entirely embracing the pregnancy, every sensation, every minute of it. I was completely in my bubble, and did not let anyone in it, really.

In January, at nearly seven months of pregnancy, we went away for a weekend of preparation for the birth (without the girls). A time for the three of us, far from everyday worries or routine. It was a wonderful retreat, down in Devon, accompanied by Olivia, who helped us so much, far more than just birth. During the weekend we did a few hypnobirthing sessions. One really struck me. Olivia let us imagine the birth of our baby as we wanted it to be. Looking back, I have the sensation, the impression, it did really go as I experienced it during that session.

We came back so relaxed, so connected to the baby: so looking forward to welcoming him or her into our family. After that, I regularly listened to my hypnobirthing cds, which had been wonderful to help me relax, and to take time for connecting to my baby. This had been really useful in helping me to find the time.

21st March, that was my presumed due date. Spring Equinox, full Moon, perfect. I was convinced it could not happen any other day. March came and went, with all the comments, everywhere, all the time: 'so still no baby?' with a surprised/worried voice. It was as if I was hiding a pillow under my coat to pretend I was still pregnant!

Gaetan, my partner, has always been very clear that he did not want a freebirth. He felt that if anything was to go wrong, he would not know what to do or how to react. He wanted to have our independent midwife in the room next door, even if she was not monitoring anything ~ no internal and no baby heart check up ~ just to have her there, 'in case'.

I have always respected his choice, and fully understand his fears.

Two weeks overdue: 3rd April

Not only did people comment constantly on it, but they also projected their own fear, their own worries onto me. Elena was very impatient to go to her friends to do the sleep-over planned for when the baby would come. I had a lot of what's called ~ so unfairly ~ 'false labour' for the previous 10 days. Our friends very kindly offered to have the girls, even though nothing was happening. We had a fantastic evening together ~ going back to the place where I shared with Gaetan ~ the joy of that new life coming to us, then to the cinema, and finally to the restaurant. We made love, not really for inducing the labour, just because we felt like it.

At 11pm I was woken up by a real pop, my water went, and splashed everywhere. My bowel emptied. I needed Rescue Remedy: could not find it. The surges where powerful and close to each other. I lit up the birth candle which had been offered to me by my friends at my Blessingway. I was already wearing the necklace we made on that day. I could not put any music on, I was already fully absorbed in the labour. I could feel my cervix open up.

11.40pm: Gaetan said to me "I am going to ring Sally" (our midwife). I thought: God you are impatient, it has only just started, it is a bit early to have her around, non? But I could not say a word, anyway.

11.50pm: Needed to go to the loo for a bowel movement. What an awful idea not to have toilets downstairs. (I made a note to have one in our next house!)

Realised on the loo that I needed to push ~ the baby that is, not anything else. The baby is coming, I want that baby to come in water. Quick, downstairs!

Gaetan opened up the pool in a blink. I jumped in it (well, as you do jump at nine months plus of pregnancy, that is). Waouhhhh, what an amazing sensation of comfort; all my muscles gave in and relaxed ~ warm water everywhere.

Just writing it, I still feel that incredible, instant sensation of total well-being ~ blissful, really: like the peace following a huge storm. At that time I knew I was in transition. I just had to fully enjoy that peaceful moment before finally having the chance to meet our baby. I felt the surge coming on. I let it open up my cervix to allow the baby glide out. One surge, the head is out. Second surge, all the baby is out ~ in water, like I have always dreamed of. We took her out of water. She was so beautiful, her eyes widely open, just looking at me. So beautiful, so peaceful, such a unique moment, just the three of us.

Sally arrived ten minutes later, with the other midwife.

This birth is everything I have ever dreamed of. It was absolutely perfect for us at that time. So empowering, and freeing. I had always listened to quick, ecstatic birth stories with envy (jealousy?), and felt so amazed. How women could give birth in only two or three hours? And here I am: Lorelie is born in an hour; freebirthed in water, just with her dad as a blessed witness.

Believe in your dreams, whatever they are. Visualise them. And believe in you, you can own it!

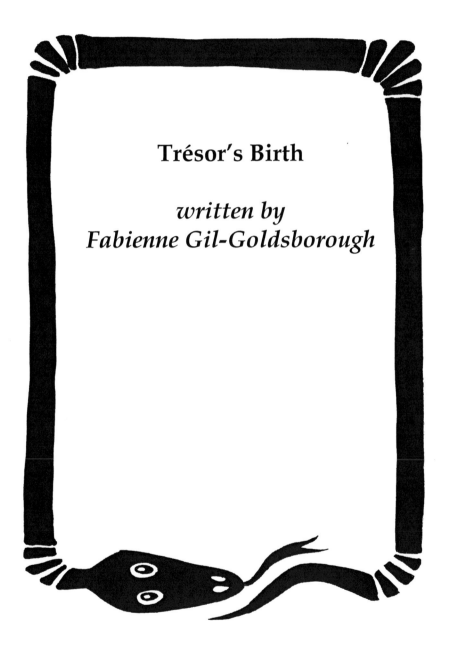

Trésor's Birth

written by
Fabienne Gil-Goldsborough

We point out that the law relating to childbirth
in the UK states that
a mother may deliver her own baby
without medical assistance.

She is unaware of this legal situation
and will need to take further advice.

As to the second point, we discuss relative beliefs
and agree to differ.

So we were going to get a visit from Social Services
and the Police
for breaking a law that does not exist.

It just illustrates that had we not known the legal position we
would have been manipulated by the system
to conform to the norm.

The following extracts from my journal tell the wonderful story of the unassisted homebirth of our second son, Trésor.

Friday, 9th August

5.00pm

I am at my friend Suzie's, when after going to the toilet, while standing up, I feel a dribble, not a wee, but water coming from the womb. I pad my pants with some tissue, but minutes later I have to go back to the bathroom, and finding a sanitary pad, I use it. I don't say a word to Suzie and the other mothers gathering in her house.

I am trying to relax and to forget about it. My husband, Dominic, is picking me up at 6pm. There is no way I can walk home. I am sitting on a chair, in the kitchen, crossing my legs, hoping to stop the leak.

Etienne, my five year old son, is having a good time playing. Dominic arrives. I feel very wet, I am wearing some jeans which fortunately can hold a lot of water without showing a wet stain as I stand up. The water dribbles down my legs, I knot my cardigan around my waist to hide my bottom, and rush into the porch to put my boots on, calling Etienne at the same time, and then rushing through the front door and into the car in a flash. As I was putting on my boots, Suzie's husband comes in, and commenting casually on the weather ~ it has been raining today ~ says "I am wet through!"

At home I feel much better.

7.30pm: I go in the lounge to rest. I am still leaking. I am a bit confused. I don't believe the labour has started. I think about my dreams of overflowing the bath, two days ago. I just dribble, dribble enough to soak four or five towels. Dominic assists efficiently. 9.30pm. We feel there is nothing happening. I go upstairs and manage to sleep.

Saturday, 10th August

I've just read Sheila Kitzinger's Homebirth. She says "if there is only a slow trickle/dribble of fluid, it is probably the hind waters, the part of the bubble behind the baby's head, that are leaking, and they often reseal themselves after a while. You can ignore it". Combined with all my dreams about overflow and false alarms, this makes sense to me. The baby is not due until the 16th of September, another five weeks. The baby is fine. I feel some kicks. I eat plenty of watermelon. Still, I don't feel like going out of the house. I go downstairs, light a candle, and ask God. His answer is simple: "Nothing is happening. Be patient." I fall asleep nicely. It's 3am.

Sunday, 11th August

The dribble is less and less. I spend my morning working slowly. It is Sunday, and I make an almond milk drink, and do some ironing and some gentle yoga for an hour before lunch. 6pm: I ring Veronika Robinson, because the leak has started again, a continuous dribble, from 4 to 5pm, wetting a pad. Veronika is very encouraging. She says that it is common for women to leak days before the birth. She suggests that I ring Sheila Kitzinger. Her phone number is in issue two of The Mother magazine.

I feel flattered to be able to speak to Sheila Kitzinger, and also nervous. She answers the phone straight away, and we talk for about ten minutes. I keep asking questions about the hind waters, with the hope that she is going to tell me that Baby will not come for five weeks. But she suggests that the labour has started, slowly but surely. She even thinks that he could come tonight. She warns me about the risks of infection, and insists that I should monitor my temperature. I know I am fine, and I have no fear of infection. I suddenly feel uncomfortable. She is the first and only midwife I have spoken to since I became pregnant, as I positively chose not to contact the medical profession. Mainly because during my first pregnancy I found that the obstetricians, doctors and midwives were all too scared about a home waterbirth, and were putting unnecessary stress on me and the baby. Now, for my second birth, I am even more confident and close to my intuition. My strong belief is that giving birth is the most natural thing in the world, and that I will be much better if left on my own. For me, this is the only way to take on all responsibility, and therefore to find within myself all the power of letting the baby be delivered.

Sheila Kitzinger seems surprised to hear that I will have my baby without the assistance of a midwife. When she enquires about how we intend to "register" the birth, she strongly advises to ring a midwife before we cut the cord (and to not cut the cord before the placenta is out), but I do not discuss that we are going to have a lotus birth. As we finish she says reassuringly "Happy Birth Day". And she gives me Michel Odent's phone number so I can get a second opinion. I am amazed to have his number, as he is so renowned in the field of home and natural birth! She adds, encouragingly, that I sound very relaxed, which I am, and suggests that I should ring Birthworks to arrange to have the birthing pool delivered tomorrow.

I now feel that I have all the information I want. I do not ring Michel Odent. I need to focus on my intuition, on my baby.

I lie down, have a shower, I have to be rested, ready mentally and physically, just in case. Dominic tidies up: last preparation, such as washing the baby bath and hanging an extra voile curtain in the birthing room. I find Etienne a little bit fidgety.

I read him a book and send him with his dad. I need to concentrate, on my own.

I rest in bed from 8pm, listening to audiotapes: chakras and meditation (Binnie Dansby).

10pm: Dominic comes to bed. He gently massages my back. I fall asleep like an angel. I wake up at 12.30 to go to the toilet, and can't go back to sleep.

Monday, 12th August

I feel refreshed. Etienne comes in bed with me. I was dry at 3am but I now have to put a pad on again. I have to plan the day by planning to do nothing. I wish I could still my mind ~ I am juggling with thoughts of "when is it going to be?"

I had another "lift" dream. The button to go up had a timer, it was very tricky for me to program it, it took me some time, and then I realised that if I stayed in the lift it would move at a very high speed, like a rewind mechanism. I decided to step out of the lift. I went up the stairs with Dominic, in our house. People from the conservatory maintenance team were waiting for us before starting their job of fixing the leak in the roof... 8.45am: Phone call from Anglian. They can come this morning, instead of tomorrow, to fix the leak on our conservatory roof! 9am: Breakfast. I need to rest. 9.45am: I write my diary. The conservatory fitters come at 11.30, and are gone at noon. I lie down a lot. I have a nap after lunch. Then I decide to ring Birthworks to try to have the pool delivered tomorrow morning. Still unsure, still confused of when it is going to happen. I ring Veronika, and my sister Marie (she had had a leak three weeks before her son's birth, but it was only a one off leak). Etienne plays in the garden. He is ever so good. 5pm: First contractions, strong. I ring Dominic to tell him that things are progressing. I feel the need to lie down. I take my clothes off. I lay on my left side, on the yoga mat, looking at the mirror. The heating is on. 6pm. Contractions get stronger. Intense. I don't move. I go into a deep relaxation. 6.30pm. For about two or three contractions I lose my focus.

I feel out of control, and instantly become aware that I have to do something or I will not be able to do this. I have to relax. My daily yoga practice helps me. I am well prepared, I am ready. The voice of Binnie Dansby then resonates in my head, echoes of an angel's voice:

Focus
Breathe
You can do it
Open your chest
Relax
Yes

I am within. I smile as each contraction goes, as we get nearer to the moment of birth. I lay, quiet, still, deeply relaxed, fixing my gaze on the mirror or on the plant. Silence. Stillness. Every muscle of my body is totally relaxed so that the uterus gets all the energy.

To the outside world my calm external appearance suggests that the contractions have stopped. Then the sensations change ~ desire of pushing. I understand that Baby is going to come out and that I should adopt another position to help him slide under me. I dare not move, as I am so deeply relaxed, any move may disturb my balance, and focus. I do it. I half squat, half sit, resting my left bottom on a cushion. On the floor is a rug covered with my yoga mat, cushioned with towels. I can see the baby's head in the mirror. The pain is far less intense than it was during the contractions. I feel completely aware and in control at this wonderful present moment. Another push or two (I didn't count, but it was quick and gentle). The baby's head slides out. I can see him in the mirror, inert, covered in white grease. A couple more nice pushes and he is born. Magic miracle. He makes some noise, bubbles coming out of his mouth. It's a boy. Small. Perfect. Beautiful. I feel so good. I rest him on my tummy, and look in wonder.

It is 8.12pm. I feel fairly energetic, not sore. I am very warm. During the contractions, I had felt very cold, I was shivering, despite the central heating and the extra gas fire heating the room, and a blanket on me. We stay on the floor for a while. Baby doesn't want to feed. The bubble noise last about 15 minutes.

Later, I feel tired in my lower back, and move on the sofa. Contractions still coming on, but more like big cramps. Waiting for the placenta. I get tired. I decide to squat to help it out.

For Etienne's birth, the third stage took four hours. It is tiring to squat while holding Baby. Back on the sofa, I get a drink of water and eat some raspberries (yummy). Three hours it takes for the placenta to emerge. It is as big as Baby. Etienne has his tea at about 10pm. Bless him.

At 11.30pm we can really prepare and enjoy our Babymoon. The placenta is in a colander, draining slowly in a big bowl. I eat a salad. Baby has latched on for the first time, at 10pm, and he has another feed in bed after midnight. I lie on my back, Baby lies on my chest. He is so little, light, asleep. I dare not move ~ to not upset him. I don't sleep much, maybe one hour. At 6.15am I ring my mum. A name? It will come later on in the morning.

It will be Trésor,
my French
golden treasure.

I feel very good. No pain. Our lotus birth Babymoon starts. On the fourth day the cord detached itself, and our baby is delivered: given to us. It is a great joy, like another birth. Wonderful first days, slow pace, love, bonding. Etienne loves his brother.

We bury the placenta in our garden, under our favourite tree.

Day nine, another chapter begins when we ring the Birth Registrar office, and the start of the stresses and strains associated with the "intervention" of the Social Services.

Intervention by Social Services

Wednesday, 21st August

Dominic, my husband, rings the Registry Office to arrange an appointment to register the birth. We know we have six weeks in which to register, but we are not hiding anything, there's no secret ~ the balloons in the front window have announced the great news to all our neighbours. The Registrar has not been notified of the birth, and so rings the local GP surgery. They have no record of any pregnancy ~ there were no pre-natal check-ups. No problem: an appointment is made.

Friday, 23rd August

The birth is registered by Dominic, who attends the Registry office alone. There are a few comments about not having medical attendance at the birth being illegal ~ a phrase we are to hear repeatedly over the coming weeks, but one we know to be untrue. In the afternoon, a midwife from the local surgery visits to see if there is anything she can do. She makes comments about the legal requirements to have a midwife present at the birth, but is otherwise very pleasant. We thank her for her offer, but decline, and she leaves. There's a message on the answer machine ~ we've switched the phone off in order not to disturb the tranquillity and harmony of the Babymoon. Mother and baby have not left the house since the birth, and we have deliberately had no visitors during this important family bonding period. The health visitor wants to arrange to come on Tuesday, after the Bank Holiday. That's fine, we know her from Etienne's younger days.

Early evening ~ someone's working late on this Bank Holiday Friday. It's the midwife. She is not as relaxed as earlier, and has clearly been in touch with some superiors. Who are these anonymous 'mysterious superiors' who will feature in the forthcoming weeks? They seem only to communicate through intermediaries. The midwife must see the baby: the Child Protection Act, Police involvement ~ are both mentioned. We agree to call back. The harmony of the Babymoon is shattered. We are very upset and worried. What are 'they' going to do? A big black cloud is forming over our heads, and the uncertainty and unknown that are forming are going to haunt us for a while to come. Nonetheless, we stick to what we believe is right, and, equally importantly, what we believe are legally our rights.

We ring back and agree that the midwife, and only the midwife, is welcome into our home to see the baby. She visits, and sees the baby wrapped in his blanket, asleep in his cot. The midwife is clearly caught in the middle, and finds the situation awkward, but nonetheless remains very pleasant and professional.

Saturday, 24th August

The local GP calls, explaining that he has been requested to attend by Social Services ~ maybe a clue as to the identity of the 'mysterious superiors'. We explain our position, our values and our motives ~ we are not against medical input where it is required, but childbirth is not an illness or injury. He is very sympathetic and civil, and outlines what examinations would normally be undertaken. We decline. He indicates that he will report back to Social Services but does not know what will happen next. We highlight that the health visitor is due to call on Tuesday. He leaves.

The uncertainty is starting to take its toll. What next? Are we all to be bundled in the back of a police van? Is someone going to take Trésor away? We dread checking the answer machine, looking in the mail box, or hearing the door bell ring ~ all our friends know not to call! Saturday afternoon ~ the duty midwife arrives, indicating that it is her legal duty to offer her service every day up to 28 days after the birth. We decline. We post a polite notice on the gate of the house indicating that mother and baby are sleeping and we do not want to be disturbed. At least that stops the doorstep calls.

Sunday, 25th August

Two messages left in the post box ~ one from the duty midwife and another from the supervisor of midwives. We read in the notes that it is a legal requirement to have baby examined, and are given a contact name and number to discuss the legal implications involving the delivery of a baby without the availability of medical assistance. We take no action. We know it is perfectly legal for a mother to deliver the baby herself without any medical assistance, whether that be in hospital or at home. The Social Services giant is either in deep thought or has decided to do nothing until after the Bank Holiday. It would be nice to know ~ we are still half expecting the dawn raid.

Monday, 26th August

The daily message is left in the post box by the duty midwife. She has been instructed to provide her legal duty to offer her service by visiting our post box on a daily basis. We have her number, so is the visit to put a calling card in our mail box really the best use of time?

Tuesday, 27th August

The health visitor comes into our home. We proudly introduce Trésor. She is the first person to see the baby since the midwife's original brief confirmation that a baby was present. She is very positive, and supportive of our choice of approach. She seems to understand our position, can see the family environment, and can see and understand the impact of the uncertainty of the position we are under. She agrees to speak with the midwife service about the necessity to visit daily, and will speak with Social Services to allay any fears and confirm that there are no welfare issues associated with the baby.

What a relief. We relax. We laugh. It's through, and the Babymoon can continue. Later in the day the daily message from the midwife appears. Disappointment. The midwife still requires an examination of the baby, and the notes in the mail box show that, despite our declining of services, the midwife is offering her service as the law requires. There is clearly a specific procedure that must be followed, and come rain or shine, that's what will be done. This will continue for another two weeks.

Wednesday, 28th August

We ring the health visitor to confirm that everything has been cleared and okayed with Social Services, and that we can truly relax. Nothing could be further from the truth. The senior social worker handling our case is writing a letter at this very moment indicating her intention to visit our home, accompanied by a police officer. Good job we just happened to ring! So the 12 hours relaxation comes to an abrupt end. The faceless Social Services machine is still trundling along. We ring the senior social worker directly. She is very pleasant, and yes, she was writing to us indicating that she would visit on Friday with a WPC. "Why?" we enquire. There's no concern over the care of the children.

The issues are:

1. We have committed an offence having the baby at home with no medical assistance (hence the involvement of the Police Child Protection Unit).

2. We have been generally irresponsible. What if something had gone wrong? (Is this the nanny state?)

We point out that the law relating to childbirth in the UK states that a mother may deliver her own baby without medical assistance. She is unaware of this legal situation and will need to take further advice. As to the second point, we discuss relative beliefs, and agree to differ. So we were going to get a visit from Social Services and the Police for breaking a law that does not exist. It just illustrates that had we not known the legal position we would have been manipulated by the system to conform to the norm. The Friday visit is off ~ just as well we called. We ask for a speedy resolution of the outstanding issues, so that we can return to normal.

Thursday, 29th August

We call again. Social Services still has no answer as to whether we have done anything illegal, and has no answer as to what the next course of action will be or what the potential consequences/implications will be. Is our child going to be taken away? Can Social Services take him away? This is not the relaxing Babymoon we desired. The issue with the Police is a separate Police matter and it is up to them as to how they proceed. We contact them directly on several occasions to determine what they are going to do. The relevant contact is unavailable, and this particular issue merely 'dies' with time. There is never any direct contact with the Police. We push Social Services for a quick resolution of the outstanding issues. We are law-abiding citizens and this 'guilty' cloud hanging over our heads is very uncomfortable. On a lesser scale, we are still pushed by the midwife to allow an examination of the mother and baby. We phone her and indicate that until the outstanding issue with Social Services is resolved we will be doing nothing. In the end, the 28-day-midwife-cover expires before resolution of the Social Services issues, so this demand effectively ends ~ it must have been important!

Friday, 13th September

Finally, we receive a letter from Social Services. A mere two weeks after we asked for an answer. Are these letters deliberately sent to arrive just in time to ruin your weekend? And in order to make up for the delay in response, we receive the same letter (with minor changes) again on the Saturday. To be hit with that sinking feeling when seeing the Social Services stamp on the envelope is not pleasant. They acknowledge the legal position regarding unassisted childbirth; however, they highlight a legal requirement to notify the birth of a baby within 36 hours, and our failure to do so (we were unaware of this requirement).

We are advised that 'Police, Senior Managers and our Legal Services Directorate ...do not wish to pursue any further action with you at this time'. However (and there was always going to be a however), they required the baby to undergo a 'new patient medical' with a GP of our choice within the next seven days, in order to be assured of no outstanding health or development issues. We responded the following day, requesting two weeks to consider the proposals, and requesting more specific details of the '36 hours notification' with which we had failed to comply (the latter never materialises).

After due consideration, and in order to resolve the matter finally, and end the Mexican stand-off, we agree to take Trésor to a GP of our choice, and initiate the arrangements on the 4th of October. The actual examination was acceptable to us as a family, and was undertaken on Thursday, 24th October.

On 19th November, a positive and pleasant final letter is received from Social Services indicating that they are happy to close their file on this matter and invite any further or outstanding questions that we might have. It has taken three months to resolve this issue and clear the air. Nobody has won.

Maybe we could have communicated more, but, as our experience showed, once you are in the system, that's it ~ irrespective of how 'right' you are.

The way things operate, it's better to stay out as long as you can ~ we knew our rights, we knew we had done nothing wrong, but that doesn't make the fight (because that's what it felt like) any easier or less stressful. Overall, I think we got off lightly. I think our Social Services (in relative terms) performed in a fairly restrained manner, but that doesn't make it right.

Some thoughts: we are in complete agreement with the role of Social Services to safeguard the interests of children, and we appreciate their requirements to investigate concealed births (as this was classified), as in some instances the circumstances (as the name suggests) may be sinister. We also appreciate that there will have been initial unfamiliarity with the legal requirements in this particular case.

In overall terms the end requirements of Social Services were quite reasonable i.e.:

a). To physically see that a birth had taken place (as done by a midwife).

b). To assess the suitability of the home environment (as done by a health visitor).

c). To confirm there were no health or development issues with the baby (as done by a GP).

However, the approach taken to reach that end point was unsatisfactory, and caused great discomfort and distress during a time which should have been very peaceful and relaxing.

1] Social Services did not have a policy for handling a planned unassisted birth. This did not conform to one of their boxes, and they seemed unable to treat it as a specific case: rather, lumping it together with sinister 'concealed' pregnancies.

2] There was no proactive dialogue with Social Services. All actions and communications came via intermediaries. It was down to us to contact Social Services. They never initiated contact, and were working from information that was incomplete: a phone call to discuss their potential concerns and how and when we might resolve these could have removed all the stresses and strains. There was no working together.

3] The legal knowledge in this area was poor, and whilst we would not expect individual social workers to be aware of the law, legal back-up should be available immediately.

4] Progress with Social Services was very slow, and there was no update on the situation or indication of where we might be going/potential consequences.

5] The attitude of Social Services came across very much as 'you are guilty, but we will let you off this time'. Maybe this works with some individuals, but someone who embarks on a planned unassisted birth should be credited with taking responsibility, and should be communicated with appropriately.

6] There was no clear indication of who was in charge of co-ordinating the various functions (midwives, GPs, health visitor).

7] Had we not been aware of our legal position we would have been steamrolled into submission by a great number of people who were quoting incorrect legal requirements.

What would we do differently if doing it again? Delay a little longer before registering the birth (so as to allow a month long Babymoon without interruption), and then arrange for the health visitor and GP to visit. This would still involve breaking the '36 hour' notification legal requirement, but unless the Social Services has a procedure in place for handling planned unassisted births, then I fear this is a price that would have to be paid. It is perfectly legal to give birth alone, unassisted ~ that is, with no midwife in attendance ~ whether this is accidental, or deliberate.

It is illegal for anyone other than a UK registered midwife or doctor to 'attend' a woman in labour, except in an emergency.

During our research the following legal requirements and information were uncovered relating to childbirth in England.

Requirement to notify birth

In the case of every child born, it is the duty of the child's father (if at the time of the birth he is actually residing on the premises where the birth took place) or of any person in attendance on the mother at the time of, or within six hours after, the birth, to give notice of the birth to the Health Authority for the area in which the birth took place. This information must be provided within 36 hours after the birth, and may be posted or delivered. This information comes from the National Health Service Act 1977 s 124 (4) as amended by the Health Services Act 1980 Sch 1 pt 1 para 75(b); and the Health Authorities Act 1995 Sch 1 para 55(b).

Any person who fails to give notice as so required will be liable to a fine, unless he satisfies the court that he believed and had reasonable grounds for believing that notice had been duly given by some other person.

Legal requirements while pregnant:
There is no legal requirement to register a pregnancy, or to attend clinics, etc., for antenatal care.

The Children Act does not cover protection of the unborn foetus, and so criminal proceedings cannot be brought in these circumstances. Unless the mother is assessed as lacking capacity under the Mental Health Act 1983, treatment cannot be forced on her, nor can her movements be restricted. A recent case may be of interest: R v Collins and others, ex parte S [1998] 3 All ER 673, [1998] 2 FLR 728. In this case, a pregnant woman refused treatment despite having a condition (pre-eclampsia) which was potentially life threatening for both her and her unborn child. She was held under the Mental Health Act 1983, and the baby was delivered. Both mother and baby survived. However, the Court of Appeal reviewed the original court decision to detain her under the Mental Health Act 1983. It was held that she was of sound mind, and, therefore, had the autonomy to make her own decision.

Care of your baby
Once a baby has arrived, he is legally a person, and aspects of his care will be the concern of others, as well as the parents. Under the Children Act 1989 s. 47 the local authority (Social Services) is required to investigate cases where there is reasonable cause to suspect that a child is suffering, or is likely to suffer, significant harm. The decision to decline an examination of a baby by a medical professional will potentially give rise to serious concern. It may be felt that in so doing, one is denying the baby the opportunity to have possible problems identified and treated. Where babies are in good health, the extent of medical intervention is fairly minimal, and families are largely left to raise their children without the involvement of the health profession, if they so choose. If one is unable to permit such involvement at any level, then one should anticipate that Social Services will continue to be involved in one's life to some extent.

Possible Social Services Intervention

If Social Services has child protection concerns, there are various ways in which it may take action:

1] Child assessment order: The Children Act 1989 s.43 (2) allows Social Services to gain access to a child for the purpose of assessing health and development, and to decide whether further action is required. It lasts for a maximum of seven days. However, Children Act guidance states that such orders should be used only where there is serious concern for the child, and not for children whose parents are reluctant to use the normal child health services.

2] The Child Protection Register: under the Children Act 1989, children's names may be placed on this register where it is felt that there is cause for concern. This is not a list of children who have been abused, but of children for whom there are currently unresolved child protection issues. Such children will be monitored by Social Services and will be the subject of an inter-agency protection plan.

3] Emergency Protection Order: A successful application under the Children Act 1989 s. 44 (4) allows Social Services to remove a child from parents on an emergency basis. It may also be used to prevent the removal of a child from hospital. Such orders may be made ex parte (i.e. without the notification or involvement of the child's parents) and last a maximum of eight days.

4] Care Order and Interim Care Order: under the Children Act 1989 s. 31, if the concerns of Social Services are sufficiently serious, they may apply to make children the subject of care orders. In so doing, they acquire parental responsibility. Although this is shared with the children's parents, Social Services has the power to override parental decisions in relation to the children. Ultimately, it gives them the authority to remove children and place them in the care of foster parents.

An interim care order is identical in effect to a full care order, but is for a limited period of time. Parents are entitled to free legal representation to oppose court applications made by Social Services.

5] Wardship: this option is little used since the introduction of the Children Act 1989. It creates a situation where the approval of the court is needed before any major decisions are taken in respect of the child concerned.

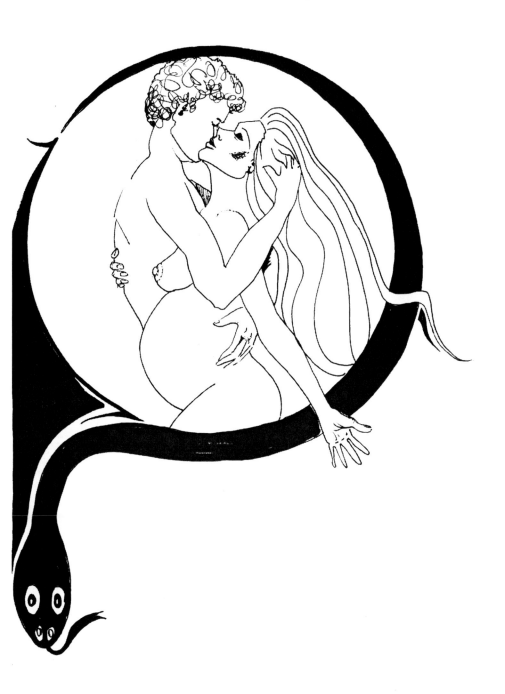

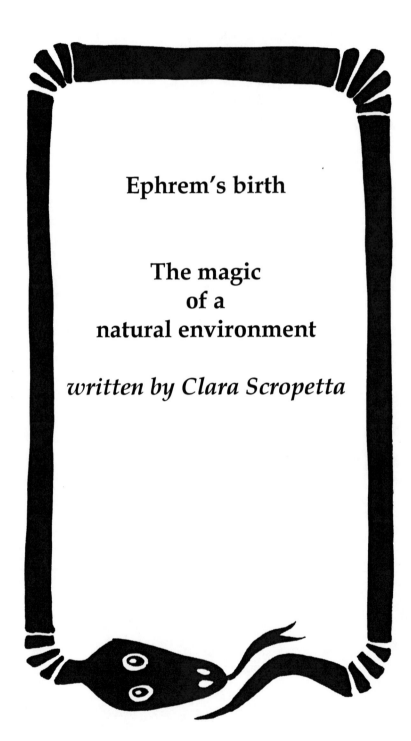

Ephrem's birth

The magic
of a
natural environment

written by Clara Scropetta

I had to find different words,
another language,
another perspective to share
what happened to me
in that special moment of my life.
I had to dive again into that
fantastic altered state of mind,
to be sincere,
accurate and incisive.

It was necessary for me to talk about it
in a different way,
touching the essence of this experience,
that had absolutely nothing to do
with measurements of any kind
(like time, dilatation, contractions)
and other practical events.
All that is outside, instead of inside.

In the clear water of the ocean

I tried several times to put this story on paper, but I was always disappointed. I was missing something, although apparently I didn't forget any detail. Then I read again the wise words of Jeannine Parvati Baker, talking about shamanic and spiritual experience (Rituals for birth, The Mother magazine, Spring 2002). I also went back to the powerful book of Vicki Noble, Shakti woman, and I understood.

My birth report was a profanation of a sacred moment. It was necessary for me to talk about it in a different way, touching the essence of this experience, that had absolutely nothing to do with measurements of any kind (like time, dilatation, contractions) and other practical events. All that is outside, instead of inside. I had to find different words, another language, another perspective to share what happened to me in that special moment of my life. I had to dive again into that fantastic altered state of mind, to be sincere, accurate and incisive. I had to forget all I read about birth, and especially all the pictures I saw. I had to distance myself from the appearance, and bond again with the real essence. So, here is the story of Ephrem's birth.

It was just the beginning of the warm season in Mauritius. Close to the full Moon, I was feeling really complete, yet I knew, within, these were our last days. I enjoyed walking every day to the little beach we chose for giving birth, and unconsciously preparing my nest: the last plants and seeds in the garden, some cleaning of the house, some letters and emails to friends.

I was feeling beautiful. I wasn't scared, I wasn't anxious. I wasn't counting, but simply living the moment. It was like I was vibrating together with this life inside me ~ we were pulsing together. I was quiet.

One early morning, under the light of a waning Moon, I discovered something jelly-like, pink, and wonderful smelling between my legs.

I went back to bed and the embracing arms of my partner, Yann-Vaï, knowing that I was going to give birth.

For several hours I ate tropical fruits, listened to the music we loved, and enjoyed loving attention from Yann-Vaï. I gave a last massage to Ephrem through my womb, under the scent of incenses and oils.

We were starting to dance together with the gentle first movements of my body, and me diving into these still unknown sensations. Like the rest of this pregnancy, I was quiet and sure. The message from Ephrem was still clear. Everything was perfect and was proceeding as it was supposed to. It was important for me to just let go, let go, accept.

Suddenly, I felt it was time, and we left for the beach with all that we thought we'd need (laugh! Now I would pack half, or even less!), with a kind of "quiet excitement". Immediately there, my 'dance' started to get a different taste. I had made a bed of leaves under a magnificent tree. It was ready, and the tree itself was decorated for the occasion with corals and shells we had collected.

Jasmine and rose incenses started to burn. I no longer talked, but was simply present for the birth.

Yann-Vaï kept on preparing the beach. He made a big fire for heating the water which we would later want for bathing Ephrem. Yann-Vaï came with me every time I wished to enter the sea and follow the waves. He paid attention if somebody was coming, and asked a few (astonished) people if they would go away. It was a cloudy, windy, fresh day. This beach was not visited much except by some fisherman, but they knew about our plan, and respected our wish for intimacy. Yann-Vaï truly protected and took care of me.

I was becoming attuned with other realities and cycles. My body was following the suggestions that were coming from all the elements. I remember well how I felt I was a kind of channel between sky and Earth: a strong ray of light and warmth was filling me, until I was simply one with All.

I felt the ground under my feet ~ soft, coral sand, and the wise life of that big tree offering support to me when I needed it. I felt the water of the ocean, full of resonance and messages, mixing with the water of the lagoon. I felt the wind.

Sea water and wind gave me movement ~ the ground and tree, stability. The sky and Earth opening, and roots.

I enjoyed the birth dance. I trusted my body was looking for what it needed: a change of position, some sea water or some tree root, a drop of ylang-ylang or a drop of Rescue Remedy.

I was moving and acting in a kind of dream, following a primal instinct. Many circles came from my pelvis. I was transforming myself into a tiger: I discovered my voice, the animal one. It was the voice of a tiger.

I was somewhere else, closer to the stars and the spirits. I remember my surprise, seeing the sun going down. I lost connection with the time. It seemed to me such a short afternoon! Suddenly, I stood up and told Yann-Vaï, "I must go in the water." I walked the few metres, separating myself from the shore. I touched, and held with my hand, the head of Ephrem coming out.

Under the glimmering light of the Moon, in the silence of the evening, the wind stayed still. Like a Queen, I entered the sea; on my knees I welcomed Ephrem, he was floating towards me, like an angel. His fantastic open eyes looked deeply into my soul. His face was full of wisdom.

It was eternity. I stood up and walked back to our bed of leaves, with this new being close to my heart, still connected to my womb through the cord.

That's the story of Ephrem being born, and it's also the story of Clara. Still a young girl, despite her age of thirty-four. After nine intense and beautiful Moons of preparation, she opened herself to experience the connection between sky and Earth. She accepted the mystery and the perfection of life. She understood her position in the Universe, finally received her missing initiation to womanhood: and she became a mother. Let's honour the silence and the mystery. Let's give thanks to the wonder of life.

Our theoretical background was the book of Leboyer, Si l'enfantemente m'etait contè (Birth without Violence). We knew nothing about Michel Odent or other spiritual midwives, we didn't even know there was a name for what we were doing: unattended childbirth. We knew nobody who had done it. We were pioneers.

The place we chose to give birth was fantastic, yet now I would look for a more intimate corner, just the next tree would have been enough. We preferred the big tree because of its beauty, but overlooked the fact that it was in the middle, open toward east. The shore offered very little sense of protection to me. We cut the cord (after it stopped pulsing, but still felt it was too early). Yann-Vaï offered Ephrem the first bath in warm sea water (without removing the casex). We went back home to find a letter from Israel with the meaning of the name Ephrem: between the sea and the Earth ~ fertility!

I give thanks to the power of Nature, and the energy of life that supported me and offered me such a magical experience.

I stood up
and walked back
to our bed of leaves,
with this new being
close to my heart,
still connected
to my womb
through the cord.

Afterword

From very early in the pregnancy, I received and accepted the message that everything was alright, and it would be possible to give birth unassisted. Me and my partner Yann-Vaï made the decision to go to Mauritius even before that, with the purpose of taking advantage of the warm, clean ocean. We had in mind a water birth because of the incredible attraction towards this element. Life is a marvellous source of suggestions. I had the privilege of visiting Flores, the most western Azorean island. In that paradise I met an Italian-French couple who had just had a baby at home. At that time I was not so much interested in all these topics; I didn't even talk really with this woman about her experience, but it was the first time I heard about giving birth outside the hospital, and I wasn't going to forget it.

At that time I was looking for novels, films, conversations, culture, so they lent me several books. Among them was one by a Portuguese writer telling the dramatic story of all the poor Azorean women who had to give birth at home with no appropriate assistance. I can't explain in a logical way, but since that time I kept a kind of seed inside me, like a subliminal imprint: clearly there was something to investigate. Not very long after, I was in Berlin visiting an exposition called Meergeboren, seaborn. I wasn't giving too much attention to all there was about birth. The exposition was generally about our relation with the sea, indeed there was something about Chris Grisgom giving birth in the sea. I remember very well lying on a water mattress listening to the whales' songs, and feeling how right it was to accept that the origin of life is in the ocean. It was like nurturing that seed I already had in me.

It was amazing the mix of these beautiful islands, full of waterfalls, volcanic lakes, powerful waves of the open ocean, with the concept of homebirth and the understanding of the origin of life.

Sure, in Flores they had a homebirth, but the fact that the place is so full of pure sweet and salt water eventually inspired me ~ and the exposition was talking not specifically about birth, but both events were a kind of reminding for me.

Of course, the angels brought Yann-Vaï to me as a lover and father, a young man of 24 who knew the work of Leboyer, and also the story of the Russian waterbabies ~ what a coincidence.

ChristoFinn's chosen birth
written by Kate Street

Graeme said he'd
never seen me look like that before,
like a goddess ~ a Turtle Goddess.

He tells people my eyes
have been changed forever.

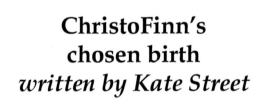

I had a wonderful, incredible pregnancy with my son. We had a powerful connection while he was in utero that I was able to strengthen with yoga, meditation, and walks in the woods. During our communications, my son guided me to the way he'd prefer to be born ~ alone with only me and my husband, Graeme. I can truly attest that this was his idea, as it's something I had never contemplated before becoming pregnant. Many times throughout my pregnancy, I thought I was absolutely crazy to even consider having an unassisted childbirth, but my son proved to be a very persuasive soul, convincing not only me, but my reluctant husband. Whenever my confidence floundered I would repeat a line I had heard in a movie,"Faith is believing in something even when common sense tells you not to", and I would find comfort.

I found my journey to unassisted childbirth to be the most powerful, freeing, and empowering experience that I have ever had.

Once I committed myself fully to freebirthing my son, I learned his name in a dream. I had asked him one night before I went to bed to tell me what he'd like to be named when he came Earthside, and all night I heard "ChristoFinn, ChristoFinn, ChristoFinn" whispered in my ear, and saw the name printed out on a chalkboard that said "Finn for short". It was so vivid it woke me up, and I was absolutely giddy. I told Graeme the next day, and we smiled at each other. Although we'd never heard the name before, it seemed strangely familiar.

I spent the rest of my pregnancy getting in my best emotional and physical shape. I dedicated myself to my daily meditations and gentle yoga sessions. I also wrote frequently in my journal to help alleviate any fears, worries, or self-doubt. I wrote a list of 24 belief statements about my impending labour that I read daily, among them that "My baby and I are fully deserving and capable of a gentle, blissful, and pain-free birth",
and "My baby will come out healthy, breathing, and maybe even smiling". When it came time to birth my baby, I felt ready. The only sign I had of impending labour was a dream the previous night of a newspaper headline reading "IT'S TIME!" And indeed it was.

I woke up at 7.00am to what I thought might be gas bubbles. But after I went to the bathroom and my "bubbles" still hadn't dissipated, I started thinking differently. When Graeme awoke, I told him I didn't think I wanted him to go to his clients' houses that day, and he looked at me expectantly and said "Really?"

We were both very excited. Around 9.30am my contractions were getting too strong to ignore ~ Graeme and I were both sure this baby would be there by noon. One of my belief statements was that I would have a short, effective labour of only five to seven hours, so that's what I had myself geared up for.

Graeme and I were having a lot of fun, joking and laughing. We made love, and it was incredibly intense and sensual. I was thinking that this labour-childbirth-thing was a piece of cake!

I set myself up in the bathroom, because I knew that's where I'd feel the most comfortable. Graeme was right there with me, rubbing my back and trying to make me laugh. My contractions, however, didn't seem to have any rhyme or reason to them.

They all seemed strong, but they weren't getting any closer together. At times, they seemed to be getting farther apart. Five hours went by, and then seven. I was already exhausted, and realised I had closed myself off by giving my labour a deadline.

Once seven hours had passed, I stopped keeping track.

It was also around then that I noticed I would have the best contractions whenever Graeme would leave the room. He would breathe with me through my contractions, and be very gentle and loving with his touch, but it seemed to be slowing me down. I told him then that I wanted to try labouring on my own for a while, and he agreed.

Graeme (who really had been very reluctant about free-birthing) surprised himself by remaining amazingly calm and peaceful throughout my labour. He let me labour alone but would check on me frequently. It was obvious to both of us, though, that I was making more progress on my own.

I had moved to the toilet to labour, thinking this was the most natural position to relax my muscles and open myself up. My contractions kept building in strength, but I really couldn't tell how effective they were. I had long ago stopped keeping track of the time, but I noticed that it had become dark outside. Soon the only light I had in the bathroom was from the three candles I had lit, and a small stained-glass turtle lamp (I had discovered after recovering from my second miscarriage that turtles were a potent symbol of motherhood and protection, and I had decorated my bathroom with turtles to prepare for this birth).

I was getting very tired, and at times, frustrated. I kept thinking I had some psychological block that was keeping me from birthing my baby. I simply tried letting everything go with my breath. While I wouldn't say my contractions were painful, I also wouldn't say they were just "intense sensations that required my whole attention" as I'd heard before. And they weren't anywhere near "blissful", as I'd been hoping. They were strong and they were very tiring. I tried lying down on the bathroom floor a couple of times when I badly needed a break, but that position didn't work for me at all. The only way I felt comfortable was on the toilet, so on the toilet I stayed, sighing loud and low with each contraction. When they would prove to be too much and too close together, I'd ask the Universe for a break "even if it meant delaying labour", and I would get a much-needed respite.

I remember at one point being intensely thankful that I didn't have a midwife or doctor with me, because even though I wasn't keeping track of the time, I knew I must be taking long enough that a professional would most likely suggest something to speed things up. I was so grateful there was no-one there monitoring me, or subconsciously pressuring me.

I alternated between too hot and too cold, and even though I was sweating, I was also shivering. I had a baby blanket over my lap that I kept removing and replacing. I couldn't eat anything except a few grapes, but I made sure to drink water after each intense contraction, and I know that helped a lot.

Eventually my strong and tiring contractions gave way to something different ~ overwhelming, body-rocking ones, that made my body involuntarily push. WOW! This was incredible! My breathing became louder and lower as I felt all the energy of the Universe coursing through my body. Now we were getting somewhere! This was a welcome change from my other contractions, because even though they were more powerful, I could tell how effective they were. I can indeed say that these awe-inspiring contractions felt wonderful!

Graeme checked in on me, as he had heard my breathing change, and I said to him "It's getting so close." He must have checked in on me ten more times, and each time I said the same thing "It's getting so close."

After probably two hours of "it's getting so close", I said to myself, "It's time to be a momma to this baby. Get him out!" I repeated that a couple of times, and I could feel my baby move down.

As I felt him moving down I said, "Okay, baby, when I feel you crowning I'm getting off the toilet."

And then he started crowning. I immediately got off, into a kneeling position. As his head started coming out I felt a burn strong enough to make me catch my breath, but it wasn't a "ring of fire" by any means. I grabbed the towel rack with the next contraction, and subsequently pulled it out of the wall. Ah, the power of birth! My husband came in when he heard the crash, and I announced "He's coming out!" Graeme offered to hold me up, but I told him I was fine, so he sat down next to me and just watched.

I reached down, and to my surprise I could feel my baby's head. It was soft and wet and wonderful! "I can feel his head!" I laughed and my baby wiggled, which made me laugh some more. I gave a push and he came out a bit more, I touched him again, and once more there was wiggling and laughter. I then said "Okay, baby, time to get you out!" I pushed, and immediately felt him coming out, "Do you want to catch him?" I asked Graeme, but he wasn't fast enough, and my baby landed softly in a pile of blankets just an inch below me.

He immediately started crying (in keeping with our deal to let me know he was breathing). I picked him up and laughed. "It's a boy! It's ChristoFinn!" Graeme beamed at me and agreed "It is ChristoFinn." I laid him gently on my forearm so he could drain anything that might need draining, and then put him to my chest. Our whole bathroom
was lit up in magic. "We did it!" I kept exclaiming, and laughing, "We did it." Our baby had stopped crying and was looking around, and then my husband saw it first, Finn smiled at us...

Graeme took wonderful photos of us, me still kneeling with Finn to my chest, covered in blood and birth. It was beauty in its most raw and perfect state. Graeme said he's never seen me look like that before, like a goddess ~ a Turtle Goddess. He tells people that my eyes have been changed forever.

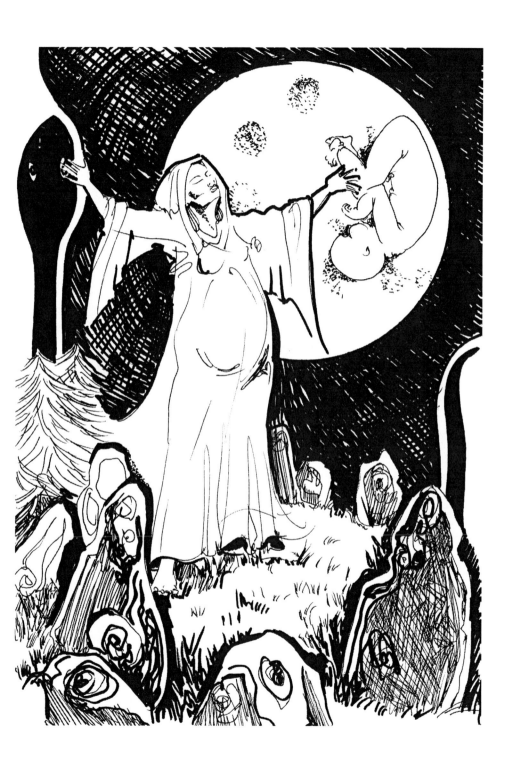

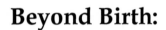

Beyond Birth:

The Quality of Birth Determines the Quality of Life

written by Julia Wilson

...all our early influences
in the womb and in infancy
are absorbed by the nervous system,
and create a behavioural blueprint
which we will carry with us
for the rest of our lives.

We all want loving and caring children. In which case, we then need to look at the roots ~ at pregnancy and birth, and the huge implications that birthing practices have on our lives, and take action ~ move away from fear and suffering towards trust and love. This was why I chose an unassisted birth for my second child.

Corin, our first child, was consciously conceived in January 2005. I went to the doctor to be checked over. Instead, we simply chatted. The doctor congratulated me, and informed me that he would put me in the system and in the next few weeks a midwife would contact me. Did he not need to check me over? I was mystified. Such a major process was taking place within me and I didn't need an examination? As I hurried back home feeling that I had wasted the doctor's time, it occurred to me that actually what was happening to me was a completely natural process. Thousands of women before me had conceived and given birth. It is not a medical problem, but an amazing experience to relish.

I trusted my body from then on, knowing that if there were problems I would be given some signs. I had a healthy pregnancy, and attended my midwife appointments and scans as I was expected to. I read What to expect when you are expecting, and some mother and baby magazines given to me by my friend, Ruth. I also went to weekly mum-to-be Kundalini yoga classes. These classes prepared me physically as well as mentally. Lucy, our teacher, taught us about the power of the breath, as well as providing us with techniques to still the mind.

As my due date grew nearer, we began to consider birth options. I knew I didn't want to be in a hospital. In a hospital, I would lose my autonomy. I would be handing my body over to others to be examined and monitored, when I wasn't even ill. Besides, the hospital was clinical, bright and strange. My husband, James, however, felt differently. He wanted me to be in a hospital so I would have a 'safe' birth. We compromised, and looked at a birthing centre. It would take 40 minutes to drive to, but if it meant I wouldn't have to be in a hospital then so be it. A few weeks before my due date, I knew instinctively that the best place for me to give birth was at home. My midwife was supportive, although she did state that I may have to go in to hospital if there were not enough midwives. I dismissed this scenario as irrelevant, as I was so determined to have our baby at home.

To even contemplate a possible complication would, I felt, cause one. James came home one day with plastic sheeting from a DIY store, so I knew that he had finally come round too. My son was born at home after a slow labour. The midwife was great. She arrived about three hours before Corin was born. She stayed in the room with me, but hardly intervened. She did examine me three times. Each time I felt disturbed, my rhythm interrupted. I felt that the extra pain I was experiencing because of these checks was unnecessary. It is only in hindsight that I can see how much these checks, as well as a stranger's presence (however friendly), slowed my labour down. Despite this, Corin's birth filled me with awe: awe of the power involved in bringing a life into the world. I felt excited by his birth and about the journey of motherhood that lay ahead of me.

When I became unexpectedly pregnant again, only eight months after having my son, I knew that I would be having this baby at home, too. I also knew that I only wanted James present. I had an easier pregnancy, experiencing little nausea and tiredness. I went back to Lucy's classes. About seven months into my pregnancy I was lent a book, Unassisted Childbirth, by Laura Shanley. She described her births so positively and fearlessly. I was inspired. I knew then that this non-interventionist birth was the kind I wanted. Far from creating fear, it actually addressed all my fears. I would be able to be at home, in my own bedroom, with no strangers examining or watching me. I jokingly mentioned it to my husband, to gauge his reaction. He would not listen, or even look at the book. A homebirth was more than enough for him, and there was no way that he was delivering a baby. He felt it was an unsafe option. I could see what he was worried about. What if there was a complication? "What if there was a complication created because of the involvement of others?" I responded. This seemed far more possible to me, given my prior experience. I knew, intuitively, that unassisted childbirth was for me, and that it was me that was going to have to get our baby out.

My waters broke gradually, beginning about 4am on March 7th, 2007. I wasn't sure at first, but the trickling was continuous, and there was no colour to the fluid, so I decided it couldn't be anything else. I woke James, and we put a plastic sheet over the mattress. James went back to sleep. I lay in bed feeling my body changing both physically and emotionally. I began to feel period-like cramps which by 7am had become unmistakable contractions.

I called Jess, a close friend, who lived nearby; she had agreed beforehand to look after Corin, (now 17 months) during my labour.

Jess arrived, and immediately began to time my contractions. She informed me they were four minutes apart. I had no idea of time, and certainly no idea that these pains were regular; however I was entirely present amidst all these intense sensations. Jess wanted us to call the midwife. I assured her there was no hurry. In fact, I was pretty close to giving birth, and I knew it. I let confidence wash over me. James left the room to dress Corin. When James returned, he called the midwife, who said she would be with us shortly. I knew our baby was on her way, and asked Jess to leave us alone. As soon as she left the room, the contractions became far more intense. I completely let go, and surrendered to this mysterious birth process. I knelt at the end of the bed each time a contraction came, circling my hips to ease the intensity. Between times I paced the floor. I felt the urge to go to the loo. I made it, and then experienced an overwhelming contraction. I felt a flicker of fear, which was quickly followed by a realisation. Only I was going to be able to get this baby out. I stumbled back to my 'spot', and began to push. This was just a physical response to the energy gathering within me. Although the urge to push became extreme, I felt the need to slow down, to pause. Part of me knew I had to do this, and I didn't question why, but just went with it. I blew out quickly, repeatedly. I then released the full force of the energy that had been building up within me. Madeleine's head was out. The phone began to ring. James went to answer it. (He later told me that he hadn't realised I was actually giving birth!) I called out for him not to as Madeleine's body slipped out and the midwife came in!

The midwife's first words were "Oh, no time for gloves", and she knelt down beside me. I felt amazing. I was on my knees as Madeleine came out, and I pulled her up to my heart.

She let out a loud cry, which surprised me ~ after all, the atmosphere was calm, quiet and dark. I felt her to find out her sex, and whispered to James that I knew as much. I'd had a vivid dream in December in which I was holding a baby girl. I was amazed by the amount of dark hair Madeleine had.

The placenta came after about 20 minutes. James gave Madeleine a bath, and then went to find Corin and Jess. I put Madeleine to my breast, and she began suckling easily. I felt so alive, euphoric, and empowered.

I had taken charge of my birth, and decided where and how I would labour. It was convenient, comfortable and safe. I was in control, and was able to experience the magic of birth without being under the influence of drugs or restrained by equipment. Ultimately, I was able to share the experience with those I love most, and to give Madeleine a calm, gentle and pleasurable welcome into life outside my womb.

Afterword

Madeleine is perfect in every way: her smell, smallness and soft breath, her warmth.

Everyone should experience the beauty and power of birth and the importance of conscious and thoughtful parenting. I have put so much into my education, my degree and my career as a secondary school teacher. It only makes sense for me now to return to the beginning to learn in depth about birth and beyond ~ not only for myself, but for my generation and those to follow.

The work of Michel Odent has captured my attention. The importance of limbic imprinting, and the influence this has on our subconscious mind and our behavioural patterns is a fascinating discovery for me. In other words, all our early influences in the womb and in infancy are absorbed by the nervous system, and create a behavioural blueprint which we will carry with us for the rest of our lives.

I have also learnt much recently from reading Sarah Buckley's book, Gentle Birth, Gentle Mothering. There is so much more research to explore. I am fully enjoying this new path of motherhood. Think of how different humankind could be if childbirth was a calm, peaceful and ecstatic experience for the majority, not the minority.

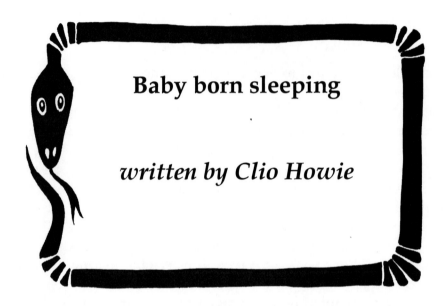

Baby born sleeping

written by Clio Howie

*I felt in tune
with the powerful energy of birth,
and felt I was the
observer rather than the participant.*

I made the decision to have Lucien at home alone after discovering Laura Shanley's website about unassisted birth. There were images of a woman laughing while giving birth in a pool outside ~ I was amazed, I never even knew that women could give birth painlessly. This awakened an interest in me about pain-free birth.

I began to research all that I could about unassisted and pain-free birth. The internet provided all the information I needed, and I used it to answer all the questions, fears and misconceptions I had about birth.

I was no longer willing just to hand over the process of my birth to doctors or midwives to be medically managed. I decided to bring Lucien into this world gently and without fear.

In the evening I had mild contractions, along with a show. In bed I would just stretch along with the contraction, and the crampy feelings would disappear. I knew my baby was on his way.

At three in the morning, one contraction lasted longer than I could stretch, and I decided to get out of bed and run myself a bath. The warm water put me into a relaxed state of mind, and I assumed I would be giving birth later in the day. I laboured with my first son for 11 hours after my water broke ~ so I was not expecting a speedy delivery with Lucien.

During contractions, I would close my eyes and go with the expanding feeling as my body prepared itself for the birth.

Suddenly, my body started to bear down, and I realised that I had entered second stage labour!

That was at half past four in the morning, and I had been in labour for one and a half hours. I called my partner, but he was asleep in bed. I had to get out of my comfortable bath and go fetch him. I told him to fill up the birth pool. He asked me to come back to bed and we would do this in the morning.

One look at the expression on my face, and he knew he had to take this seriously!

We had prepared and practised in the pool, and it was already inflated. I knew that if I wanted to have Lucien in the birth pool I would need to get in as soon as possible. When it was deep enough, I climbed in, relaxed, and let the birthing process begin. I did not push. I stayed calm, and was rewarded by having no pain at all. I felt my tissues expanding, and I accepted the process instead of trying to fight it. I felt in tune with the powerful energy of birth, and felt I was the observer rather than the participant.

I allowed my body to push without any conscious effort on my part. I felt inside the birth passage to touch the crinkly roundness of my baby's fuzzy head. He had come lower down, and I felt anticipation for his arrival.

During one of the pushing sensations, Lucien's head appeared and then disappeared. The next contraction presented his head fully. The cord was wrapped twice around his head. I felt under the cord to see how tight it was ~ it was easy to slip my finger underneath, but not loose enough to go over his head. I confirmed this with my partner, and we decided to leave it until he was born.

Lee told me that Lucien's head was rotating. I witnessed the beauty of Lucien's face beneath the water, in the next contraction he was out. I lifted him to my chest, and unravelled the cord from his neck and body.

He was so peaceful, and seemed asleep. I gently rubbed and patted his back to see if he was alright. He crooned softly, and snuggled closer to my breast. I blessed him with his first kiss.

Lucien was born surrounded by the love of his family, under dim candle light, and in a quiet room.

His first experience was to be held gently in the waiting arms of his loving mother, with timelessness as a companion, and the first joy of tasting the sweet milk from his mother's breast, uninterrupted. Happy birthday, Lucien. May love always be the path that follows you. Lucien Blaze was born on the 30th of October 2007, at 5am.

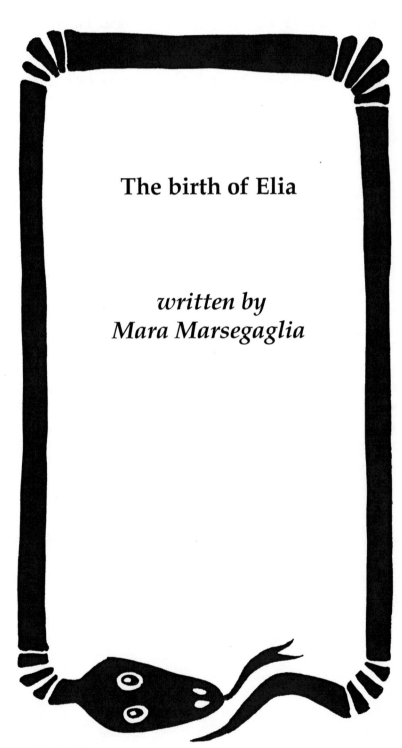

The birth of Elia

written by
Mara Marsegaglia

The day of your coming was near. We knew it. Long walks in the forest made waiting nicer. I remember visiting the immense beech tree, imposing and ancient, with its large branches embracing and reassuring us. That night I felt something stirring in my womb. I woke Claudio to tell him you might be coming soon. We looked at the clock, and it was four. That sensation, together with a light pain, came back again at short intervals. That was how the beginning of labour had been described to us, and I started to let myself go and listen to my body. We remained in our bed until dawn, trying to rest. Then a big hot Sun came and called onto the terrace.

We prepared the place where I felt I would open myself for your birth: beside the stove, the window and the sofa. However, we stayed on the terrace for the whole morning, lying down on a blanket in the sun. Standing up, sitting down ~ trying to follow your descent with soft and round movements, breathing deeply. Claudio was there. In front of me. Behind me. Next to me. Listening. Hugging. Supporting. Cuddling. Then something invited me to return to our nest to rest on the sofa. I asked Claudio to light the fire, and I continued to listen to my body, and adopted positions that could enable your journey. Crouched or standing; when my legs were tired I lay on my side. I went to the loo and threw up several times. My body was clearing itself. Claudio brought basins, cleaned me and the space around me, encouraging me. The contractions were increasing in intensity and frequency, with unexpected power. Your head was pressing on the bottom of my back as you were going down. It was opening the way. Meanwhile, the Sun had gone and the darkness was slowly enveloping us. Claudio lit a candle. I crouched, without knowing that soon you would come. Then I got down on my hands and knees. Claudio was behind me. He checked if and how much I was opening. I felt the roundness of your head with my hands. At a certain point my waters broke, spilling out a warm liquid. Now there were no membranes to keep you separated from the world outside; and I was able to feel your hair, fine and wet. Now the door was opening. Strong, soft and elastic. I felt Claudio would look after you and sweetly welcome you. Your tiny head came out first. Your eyes were open, Claudio tells me. Some liquid came out from your nose and mouth, then you screwed up your eyes with a pained look. 'Push, Mara!' I pushed, and you slid out. First a hand, then your shoulders and legs. Claudio asked me to lie down so that he could join us in an embrace.

Small and slippery. A short moan. Your breath on my heart. First I felt you; I was not looking at you straight away. We looked at the clock: it was six, on a warm Autumn afternoon. Outside were Autumn leaves, and the voices of the inhabitants of our little village. Later, the placenta came: your travelling companion. We placed her next to you, and watched you both for a long time.

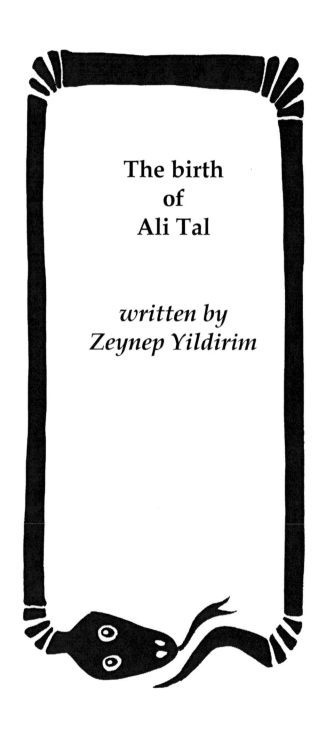

The birth
of
Ali Tal

written by
Zeynep Yildirim

The room, lit with a candle,
was a temple filled with prayers
pronounced by me
and humans of other
places and times.

I didn't know them,
but I could feel their love.

I closed my eyes
to surrender to the journey.

I have tried so many times to write this article. It is hard to describe with words what happened during birthing. My body cracking up, the mind in hypnotic, deep contemplation; the gentle mammal in me issued forth. I felt totally part of Nature for the first time ~ together with all women, sisters, mothers, Goddesses of all times, and newborns of all species.

Both my pregnancies triggered huge transformation, channelled by my intuitive desires. My first daughter called me out of the city life into the woods, and my second pregnancy guided me into sensible introspection. I have further been touched and deeply transformed by my experience of motherhood. Nevertheless, I felt the power of being a mother for the first time inside my own hands, when I caught Ali coming out of my body. I was alone to give birth. When ready, Ali initiated his journey down, and I patiently let it happen. I closed my eyes and felt touched by the Divine. I was in deep meditation, that which was happening was bigger than myself, and I remained humble in the midst of the hardly bearable intensity and the state of altered consciousness.

I also wanted to give birth by myself to my first child, Peri. Life had already suggested to me unassisted birth. I first heard the story of Ephrem's freebirth. I remember feeling so grateful to receive the information that it was possible. That story put a seed in me which has led me to reclaim my humanness, my freedom to follow my heart. I followed other signs before and during pregnancy, but I didn't yet trust life enough to know that when you humbly accept not to be in control, even if sometimes things seem to go wrong, then surprisingly gorgeous things happen. When I look back, I don't understand how I could trust a midwife more than myself, and life itself. And I sadly remember thinking, in the middle of labour, "Why is this stranger here in my bedroom, during this most important and intimate event of my life, telling me what to do? She doesn't love me, and doesn't really care what I feel or what happens to me." I lived her interventions as abuses, and felt afterwards, that my childbirth experience had been stolen from me. Nevertheless, there still had been long hours when I was alone with my baby and my faith, and things were the way they were. It was a shamanic experience, of surrender and awakening to universal consciousness. I felt one with my baby and with All That There Was. I saw eternity in my baby's eyes when I first looked at her.

That's why, the second time, I chose to give birth all by myself; there was to be no mental noise from the thoughts of other people: only the Great Mystery that I embraced. I was alone, but I was not separated. I loved life, tried to live it as well as possible, and loved my partner, even though I was yet unsure of my ability to love. I conceived consciously, and did no tests on my body through pregnancy. I addressed my doubts and questions directly to my baby. I listened to my dreams. I walked in the woods, and talked to the sea. There was nothing but my babies, my partner, my friends, Nature and all. I enjoyed every moment of pregnancy and birth. I had no fear and felt no pain.

I started to lose my waters one morning, and kept losing a little bit of water at a time all day long. It happened to be an exceptionally warm November day, and I thought the beach would be an excellent place for my waters to pour down my legs. I made it a lazy day on the beach, laying down on the rocks, either sleeping or listening to the waves. My family joined me for lunch with a basket of food freshly bought at the farmers' market, and they left me alone again after lunch. They all seemed happy and excited, yet calm. I saw them later again for dinner in the house. Everyone pretended it was a normal day, yet they were touched by the magic. I don't have much memory of that dinner. My contractions started when I retired to our bedroom, just after dinner. I squatted on the floor. The room, lit with a candle, was a temple filled with prayers pronounced by me and humans of other places and times. I didn't know them, but I could feel their love. I closed my eyes to surrender to the journey. The contractions started slowly. I called Jeremy, and convinced him to ask everybody to go sleep in their rooms, in order to leave me and the house in peace. I came out of the room a little later, attracted by the huge and beautiful fire that Jeremy had made. The crescendo of my contractions became one with the fire, and I remained there, squatting on the floor, holding on to the sofa. I got lost in the warmth, filling everything that surrounded me. I was a Priestess in trance, and I felt not alone: there was the tribal music of the crackling fire, and the dance of its rays. I perceived the increasingly intense contractions amidst the alchemical blending of elements of all sorts. The fulgurate dance of the fire was topped by a calmness emanating from inside me, from Ali.

Some time later, Peri came in crying, with Jeremy. I wanted to breastfeed her, but it made my contractions feel painful.

Jeremy prepared a warm bath. Peri and I both got in. The water absorbed me immediately, and I closed my eyes again, to start a primitive song. Peri and Jeremy stayed there watching me for a while, with astonished eyes, until Peri fell asleep in his arms and they both turned back to sleep in the room. My song continued the whole time I was in the bath. The warm water felt so good, as if my body sweetly melted into it, as if I had been there forever. I was comfortably feeling Ali making his way down the waters of my birth canal. When he arrived all the way down, I touched myself and felt his hair on my fingers. I felt agitated, I opened my eyes, looked around, and felt cold. I went and sat on the toilet to poop. I had a sudden thought of death, but it didn't scare me. Everything was so perfect, pure, untouched, unaltered, that I accepted it, and it vanished. Then I made it to the bidet, and felt a primal urge to push. After three intensely pleasurable pushes, I got up and caught Ali. There he was, in my hands, his eyes looking into my eyes, telling me all the love there was. I thought "we made it". It was unbelievable, yet felt so real inside my hands. I knew him, I didn't need to look at his genitals to know he was a boy.

He was Ali of my dreams. I felt like crying, but I could only smile, our eyes locked together in the silent dark. After a while, I wanted to share the news. I called Jeremy and Alice. They greeted Ali, who was already suckling at my breast. They helped us to move near the radiator, where I pushed for a last time for the placenta. Then they prepared a bed next to the fireplace, and I spent all night looking at my baby and feeling the sacred, the perfect, the eternal he was emanating. Peri woke up another time and joined me for a breastfeed. When she saw Ali, she said with surprise "What's this, questo?" [I am Turkish, but lived in France, California and Italy. My daughter, Peri, 3 years old, knows all these languages. Indeed, generally she doesn't speak Italian to me]. I said "It's a baby."

She was so excited, she touched and observed the "piccole mani" [little hands] and the "piccoli piedi" [little feet]. And we stayed there, with the fire, its rays dancing on the walls, all of us making silence, touched by the otherworldly essence filling up the whole room. Alice and her children woke up with the sunrise. They were enthusiastic to meet the baby. I said "This is Ali's first sunrise." The sky put his most intense red colour up, and then filled the room with amazing light.

My friend Clara arrived that morning, just as we planned, except that she didn't get the message I sent on the phone the previous day, telling her that Ali was on the way. She just woke up and felt like packing to come to our house. When she entered the room, a special smile covered her face, and she said "mais il y a un bébé ici [but... there's a baby here]," intuiting what happened, before having seen the baby.

She had met the family on the porch, they said hello, but kept silent about the birth. She took care of me impeccably, the placenta, the house, the kitchen, the children, the relations and the postpartum emotions. Our Babymoon was not of the most intimate ones, with more than a dozen people in the house, but I felt at home with my big family. All, including the youngest ones, were conscious of the sacredness of the event, taking delicate care of me, and making space for us to rest and to know each other.

I believe a woman who has given birth by herself can only desire to nurture her babies, to cultivate her woman-ness and to give more birth: that which makes her woman.

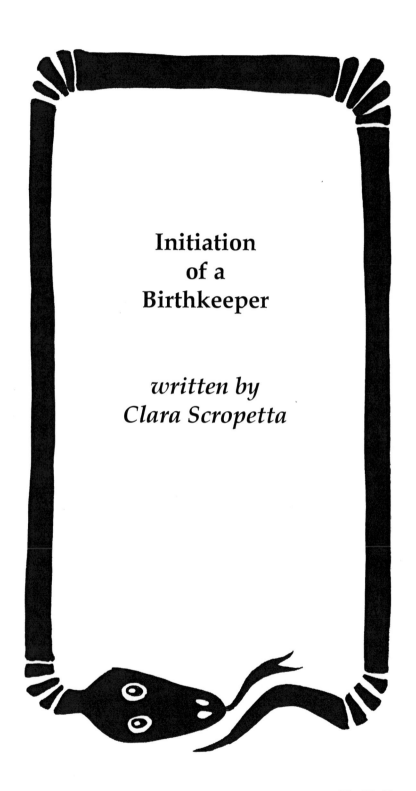

Initiation
of a
Birthkeeper

written by
Clara Scropetta

When I met Sara the first time, she was already pregnant. She was beautiful. She told me she hadn't done any exams or check-ups; I felt she did them spontaneously. She felt good, and knew that everything was going right.

However, she didn't know yet where she would prepare her nest, and she didn't want to see the father of her child. She said she was not in love with him. She told me a meaningful dream, which I don't remember now, but at that moment I thought it was a good omen. It was July. Some days later, I discovered that I knew the father, Simone. He wished to be there for this child, and was waiting, trustful that she would change her mind. I saw them getting closer at the end of July, just a little bit. Felice, Simone's father, said: 'She really doesn't want to have anything to do with him,' and I said: 'In any case, you will become a grandfather.' Simone's mother said: 'Things will go right; I'll become a grandmother, anyway!' I saw them at the end of September ~ Sara, even more florid and beautiful: Simone, smiling and enthusiastic. The nest would be at Felice's home. I promised her I would be there just after the birth, if she wished. We didn't talk much on that occasion. She continued to feel good and confident, to receive meaningful dreams. She continued to enjoy the spiritual contact from the child in her womb.

In November, I wrote a short letter, to support and encourage them. I knew they intended to welcome the child unassisted. Sara came to me, and was even more beautiful then the last time. They explained to me that they decided to come out of respect to Felice. He didn't feel comfortable thinking of an unassisted birth at his home.

A couple of days later, we looked for a suitable place so they could prepare their nest. Then, there would be no other obstacles at the end of the pregnancy. However, Sara didn't feel serene. Several people talked to her about the fact that she'd had no exams or scans, so she was not sure if everything was right: about the shape of her womb; would the child remain in a breech position? Would it be better to turn him, or ask for assistance? Sara came and talked to me. She felt downhearted.

We called a meeting in the community to talk about the intention of Sara and Simone to give birth here. It soon became a cathartic circle of choral liberatio: fears awakend from the determination and clearness of Sara.

Words like responsibility, safety, risk and suchlike made me start every time ~ Sara could have been me, when the birth of Ephrem was near and I had the intention of doing it by myself! At the end, the consent went to unconditional support and full trust. Sara and Simone finally had a home and a solid human surrounding.

Sara ended her spiritual isolation and went back to community life; the sun kept on shining. I had no reason to doubt that everything would be perfect.

I left for a week-end, and when I was back, Sara came and looked for me. She had been in labour for two days and two nights. She was tired, exhausted. I hugged her, listened and gave support. I let her drink some water. I took my smallest child, Taro, with me and went with her. Simone was preparing a hot bath.

While we walked there, some people followed us (they were already with her, before I was back). In the room upstairs there were seven people, plus the baby in the womb. I wished I could tell somebody to leave, but ~ luckily ~ Simone did it for me. Good, two people less. There were still too many however, and some people talked and asked too much of Sara. I kept silent. I gave her a drink. I lit incense. I asked Spirit what to do. I wished to create a space where Sara could feel safe and was not disturbed, but at the same time I didn't want to impose myself on anyone.

Everyone was offering gifts. It was just a question of harmonising. The bath was ready. There were still three of us, in addition to Sara and Simone, and it was so hard to have a bit of silence. Sara relaxed in the water. Her body warmed up. I kept giving her drinks. Water, lemon and honey. For two days she had barely eaten. I wet her face with warm water, and caressed her. My gestures were calm and confident; inside me the energy of trust and patience grew. I looked at her and instinctively turned towards Simone: 'She's so beautiful!' He nodded.

From this moment, the atmosphere changed and became more intimate. Words rarefied. First Jeff, then Imma, left the room; they had given strength and support. Now we could continue in silence and peace.

At a certain point, Sara asked: 'Is it ok to push, if I feel like it?' Smiling, I answered: 'What you feel is what you need in that moment. Nobody else knows better than you.'

I felt she had gained strength and she was again connected to herself. I felt she was letting herself go.

A light and an otherworldly power radiated from her. She slept at intervals, for a very few precious moments. She was beautiful, radiant. The bath came to an end, and we went back to the room. Everything was alright. I caressed her womb. The child was big and had his back on the left. Sara asked if it was normal; without a word, but with a smile, I showed her the movement the baby would keep doing: down like a spiral.

I nodded off in a corner of the bed, Taro on my side, close to the two/three of them, while labour went on. Slow, but powerful. Sometimes Sara looked for my hand; I held her and caressed her womb. At a certain point she said: 'The child is still high.' After a moment, I asked: 'Does he feel high?' 'Yes.' 'And what is stopping him from coming down?'

Sara was a little bit nervous: 'I don't know! You tell me!'. I surprised myself, telling her confidently: 'Nothing.' She didn't want anything, but asked: 'I haven't got contractions now, should I push?' Resolute, I answered: 'It's not necessary to do anything, everything comes by itself, be patient.' Time passed, dilated itself. Some contractions came, but they were not enough. And time kept dilating. I walked up and down, cradling Taro, hypnotically; and time went on dilating, till I started doubting. In my head, terrible questions came: is it the umbilical cord? Is it the shoulder? Should I do something?

I asked the flame of the candle, and the answer came to me strong and clear ~ 'This child feels good, and wants to come slowly.' I turned towards Sara with a smile on my face and in my heart, again full of that same faith that, till then, hadn't abandoned me. From that moment the head began to appear, enveloped in membranes. The labour went ahead slowly. It took ages to proceed, I didn't know how many times this little head went up and down. Many, so many times, until it emerged completely, without going back any more. We could breathe life ~ it was transforming itself. The air was so impregnated with it, that even Taro woke up, even though it was the middle of the night. Sara was radiant, and Simone, quiet and trustful.

In that moment, Sara, beautiful and strong, on hands and knees, stood only on her knees, and the child came ~ so suddenly that he fell on the bed. The hands of his parents, together, took him and brought him to his place, in Sara's arms, against her breast. He cried for a moment to get rid of the mucus.

Sara sucked on his mouth a few times to free it. A beautiful, big baby, well-grown, perfect. Rosy, calm, warm, he started to breathe. Placid, his eyes well open.

Even his head was only a little lengthened, I think because the waters broke at the last moment. No meconium. Sara didn't tear. What wonderful moments, in absolute calm and silence. What a blessing. The candles lit us, silence enveloped us. Sara and her baby had a warm bath, and then, in the bed, the placenta arrived. Whole, big, healthy. I looked for a basin to put it in during the night. I made sure that Sara and her child were well covered and warm, that she had something to eat and drink, and, with an immense joy in my heart, I closed behind me, the door of their room.

The day after, Imma (the other woman who was present in the evening), imagining that the baby was born during that silent night, opened the door and entered Sara's room, looked inside the blanket that covered mother and baby, and was astonished: such a big baby! She had never seen one that size before. Imma is a mother of five, and has been at about one hundred births in the community.

Tiglio (lime-tree), his name, first son born of Sara and Simone. As regards the impact of an undisturbed birth on the mother's behaviour, I can affirm that seldom have I seen a lioness like Sara was, and still is.

Two weeks after birth, she told Simone, who asked to take the baby for a walk while she had a rest: 'No way! Of course, you can hold Tiglio, but you can't go anywhere with him. What if he needs me? He has to stay close to me!' Many in the community accused her of being too egoistical, because she felt good holding Tiglio, and she didn't want to give him away. Oh, I pray for people to be moved to tears by the vision of a mother with her baby in-arms, and never, ever blame her for that. Blessed be, the voice that guided me to be faithful and patient! A woman asked to give birth naturally, with her strength, on her own. It was exactly like that, even if she wasn't alone the way she expected. A child was born in peace and love, in his way, and at his pace. I was called to keep the purity and the integrity of the place, to keep away fear and agitation. The Spirit nourished me, and guided me in all my gestures and acts, offered with grace and thrift. I did nothing, almost. This initiation as a Birthkeeper was a very big gift. I'm so grateful...

Facts and figures for those who want to know:

Labour began on Friday, during the day (morning).
By Saturday afternoon labour wasn't effective any more.
Saturday, 10pm, labour started again.
The baby's head appeared at 2am.
The baby's head was completely outside at 3.30am.
The rest of the body followed at 4am.
No-one checked Sara during pregnancy or birth.
From Saturday evening to the birth, Sara asked me four questions in eight hours!
The head of Tiglio was outside for half an hour, at least, before he was completely born!
Tiglio was lotus born three days later.

By the way, this year, at a women's gathering, Sara spoke about how she'd been very impressed by a positive comment. When we first met that Saturday evening, she explained to me what happened in those two days, adding that several people were very concerned about this strange birth. I told her, 'It's not a strange birth, it's your birth! If mother and baby are fine, everything's fine. Let's keep mother and baby fine.'

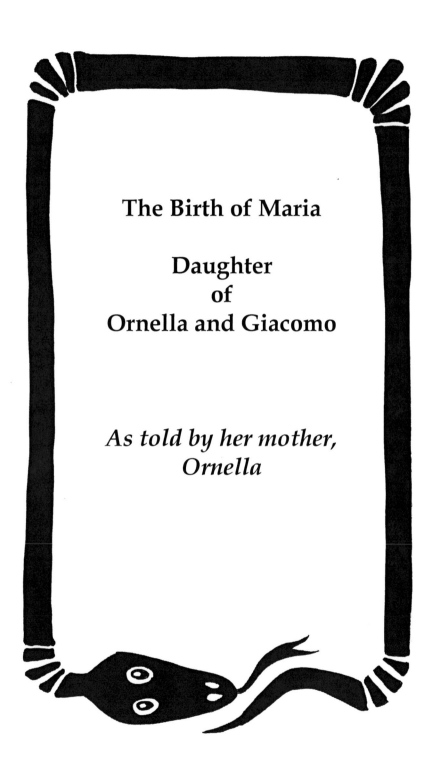

The Birth of Maria

Daughter
of
Ornella and Giacomo

*As told by her mother,
Ornella*

In a dream,
around the sixth month of pregnancy,
I was near the coastline,
a stormy sea with high, powerful waves;
a friend asked me when I would give birth,
and I answered
"The 22nd of July."

I remember that night, when my partner Giacomo and I made love gently while sleeping (the morning after, I left for Castiglioncello, to attend a congress about midwifery art, a topic very dear to me), our bodies lying one above the other, before we surrendered softly to sleep again. I whispered without thought or intention, "Here's Maria." Almost dream-like, pronounced lightly, without coming out of my mouth, inserted like a diamond between the smiling lips.

So Maria revealed herself, and I welcomed her into my womb. To tell about the conception of Maria is indissoluble from her birth, and from the nine months I cherished her in my body. Maria came to light on the 22nd July, at dawn, amidst the simmering of the countryside surrounding our home, after a night with strong wind, moanings, fragrances, silences filled with breathings.

July 22nd. In a dream, around the sixth month of pregnancy, I was near the coastline, a stormy sea with high, powerful waves; a friend asked me when I would give birth, and I answered "The 22nd of July." The revelation of her name, of her sex, of her birthday, are just a few strong signals with which that daughter of mine talked to me. I kept them with attentive consciousness. The respect I nurture for the mystery, the "ungraspable", the imponderable made it impossible for me to declare so confidently that I would give birth in a certain way, instead of... but I wove day after day, while she was growing in my womb, the framework that led me as far as that night, when contractions started, and I felt, with absolute certainty, that I wouldn't call anybody. No assistance, no people.

Looking after me was a candle, lit around midnight, to whom I confided that, before it burned to the end, I would give birth. It happened right around midnight, that our waters started, drop by drop, to run down my thighs. It seemed to me blessed water ~ it was very scented and made me feel good. At home, everybody slept: my first born, Niccolò, 7 years old; my nephew, Filippo, 6 years old; and my partner, who reassured me before going to sleep, saying: "I'm here, if you need something, you just have to call me." His presence was so important to me. He was the masculine energy that didn't watch, didn't interfere, indeed was simply there, present in the air. I took my place in the kitchen, in front of the fire, with an old futon, an excellent Brazilian incense and my candle. It started, the slow and inexorable dance of contractions, which, one after the other, like sea waves, came and opened me, more and more.

I took my place in the kitchen,
in front of the fire,
with an old futon,
an excellent Brazilian incense
and my candle.

Sometimes, there was a light resistance in me towards that opening, towards letting life pass through me in all its impetus, because life, sometimes, is so strong it shakes you. Nevertheless, I never doubted that something wasn't going the right way, I felt my body in its whole integrity; I perceived every nerve ~ owner and servant of what evolution wisely conserved. I walked, I squatted. Slowly, my moanings were transformed into a song, a rhythmic voice exercise, a cyclic lullaby. Outside the window, the wind was shaking the trees; then I realised that it was close to dawn. The song became a panting silence, I was completely naked. I caught an Indian tissue, and I arranged it around my head to form a turban, a gesture that gave me strength. I said "Beloved, it's dawn. It's time to be born, your Mama is here." It was the first time I talked to her with words, even though for nine long months we enjoyed an inner dialogue. Then my voice was transformed into a deep cry, like it was emerging from a mountain cave. Then silence.

The head came out, and my hand, gentle and ready, lightly touched her. I felt it slightly rotating, and I was in awe in front of such a new and such a wise movement. A moment after, she slipped out between my arms. Maria came into the light ~ immense joy, amazement, shivering, infinite love.

Maria latched on straight away at the breast, to suck her precious nectar. Her eyes wide open, she stared at me while feeding, and fed for hours and hours. Shortly after, the placenta was born ~ wonderful, scented, pulsating: no intervention, a natural lotus birth.

Myself, Maria and the placenta spent four days embraced, shrouded with light and fragrance.

Maria, now, is here in my arms, and smiles very much. Some will say it's only a reflex, but I know that she's smiling to life. This birth is dedicated to my whole family; to midwife Carla Joly, with whom I danced and meditated in the pregnancy months, who never stood in my way or failed to support me in my choices, and who, wisely, was able to let me be alone; to Clara Scropetta, Birthkeeper, whose presence I felt fluttering in my house that night; and to all those who haven't enjoyed an undisturbed birth.

Author's Notes

Pregnancy, birth and parenting practices amongst tribal women:
For all references related to our ancestresses in regard to pregnancy, birthing and postpartum, I have drawn upon Judith Goldsmith's seminal work ~ Childbirth Wisdom from the world's oldest societies. This huge study brings together evidence from 500 tribal cultures around the world.

Essential oils in pregnancy and birth
Balacs, Tony: Safety in pregnancy, International Journal of Aromatherapy 4, no. 1 Spring 1992; 15.

Women designed to deliver their own baby
Childbirth Without Fear by Grantly Dick-Read.
Evolution's End by Joseph Chilton Pearce.

Intravenous vitamin K has been linked to childhood leukaemia
Golding J., Paterson M. and Kinlen L. Factors associated with childhood cancer in a national cohort study. Brit. J Cancer 1990;62:304-8.
Greenwood R. Vitamin K and childhood cancer. MIDIRS 1994;4(3):258-9.
Greer F., Marshall S, Cherry J. and Suttie J. Vitamin K status of lactating mothers, human milk, and breastfeeding infants. Pediatrics 1991;88(4);751-6.
Meyer T. and Angus J. The effect of large doses of Synkavit in the newborn. Arch Dis Child 1956;31:212-5 in, Ruby, C. Vitamin K: a historical perspective. MIDIRS 1997;7(3):362-4.
Hall M. and Pairaudeau P. The routine use of vitamin K in the newborn. Midwifery 1987;3(4):170-7
Hathaway W. New insights on Vitamin K. Hematol Oncol Clin North Am 1987;1(3):367-379.
Golding J., Greenwood R., Birmingham K. et al. Childhood cancer, intramuscular vitamin K and pethidine given during labour. BMJ 1992;305 (6849):341-6.

Homebirths safer than hospital births
In his book, The Five Standards for Safe Childbearing, David Stewart, PhD, asserts that every 29 minutes a baby dies unnecessarily in US hospitals.
Mayer Eisenstein, MD, The Home Court Advantage, 1988.

The five post birth needs of every baby
Evolution's End by Joseph Chilton Pearce

Autism and early life factors
Birth and Breastfeeding by Dr. Michel Odent
Primal Health by Dr. Michel Odent

The legality of unassisted birth in England
www.aims.org.uk/homebirthUpdated.htm

Recommended Resources

www.ucbirth.com
Consultations with Laura Shanley, author of Unassisted Childbirth
Are you pregnant and planning an unassisted or midwife-assisted
homebirth, but still have apprehensions? Or are you recovering
from a home or hospital birth that was less than ideal? I provide
loving, non-judgmental support, education and encouragement to
both women and men, either in person or over the phone. For more
information, or to schedule a session, please visit my website –
www.ucbirth.com/consultation.html, write to me at laurashanley@
comcast.net, or call 303-521-5848 (USA, Mountain Time Zone).
Laura Shanley is a writer, author, mother and birth consultant in
Boulder, Colorado, USA
www.detoxyourworld.com
Your one-stop shop for all ethical and vegan supplements, super-
foods and conscious eating requirements. It stocks Nature's Living
Superfood, Maca and vitamin C (made from cherries).
www.greenlife.co.uk
Green Life Direct stocks liquid vitamin B.
www.ifer.co.uk
International Flower Essence Repertoire for essences from around
the world.
www.ecstaticbirth.com
This educational childbirth site is brilliant. Contact Binnie Dansby if
you wish to receive Breathwork. I recommend Binnie's Breathwork
without reservation.
www.united-chiropractic.org
To find a chiropractor in your area.
www.birthkeeper.com
Website dedicated to the work of the late Jeannine Parvati Baker.
www.sarahjbuckley.com
Dr. Sarah Buckley is the author of Gentle birth, gentle mothering.
www.waterbirth.org
International waterbirth information centre ~ acts as a clearing
house for waterbirth research and studies from around the world.

www.ttfuture.com
(Brilliant resource, and references to all the work by James Prescott
PhD, as well as Joseph Chilton Pearce and Michael Mendizza). Creating optimal growth and learning environments.
www.lovefrombaby.com
Beautiful birth cd, and Messages from the womb meditation cd (these
were created by Birthkeeper, Kate Street).
www.themothermagazine.co.uk
International magazine on holistic and conscious parenting ~ from
pre-conception throughout childhood (founded and edited by
Veronika Robinson).
www.compleatmother.com
American publication on natural pregnancy, birth and breastfeeding.

Recommended Reading

Childbirth wisdom by Judith Goldsmith
Unassisted childbirth by Laura Kaplan Shanley
Evolution's end by Joseph Chilton Pearce
Magical child by Joseph Chilton Pearce
Childbirth without fear by Grantly Dick-Read
The continuum concept: in search of happiness lost by Jean Lieldoff
Primal birth by Dr. Michel Odent
Birth and breastfeeding by Dr. Michel Odent
Birth without violence by Frederick Leboyer
Prenatal yoga and childbirth by Jeannine Parvati Baker
Hygieia: a woman's herbal by Jeannine Parvati Baker
Conscious conception by Jeannine Parvati Baker
Messages from water by Masuaru Emoto
Fathers-to-be handbook by Patrick Houser
Parenting for a peaceful world by Robin Grille
The biology of belief by Dr Bruce Lipton
CALMS: a guide to soothing your baby by Carrie Contey and Debby Takikawa
Lotus birth by Shivam Rachana
Fresh vegetable and fruit juices by Dr. Norman Walker
The natural way to vibrant health by Dr. Norman Walker
Breast milk: a natural immunisation by Joanna Karpasea-Jones
Comparing natural immunity with vaccination by Trevor Gunn
A compendium of flower essences by Clare G. Harvey, Peter Tadd, Don Dennis
Everybody's guide to homeopathic medicines by Stephen Cummings and Dana Ullman
Sleeping with your baby: a parents guide to co-sleeping by James J. McKenna
Conscious eating by Dr. Gabriel Cousins
The power of now by Eckhart Tolle
A new Earth by Eckhart Tolle
The Ringing Cedars of Russia series by Vladimir Megré
You can heal your life by Louise Hay

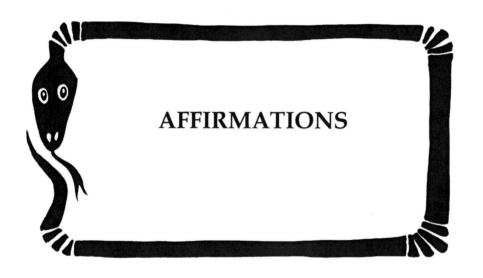

AFFIRMATIONS

On the following pages are affirmations you can use throughout pregnancy and birthing. Take time to meditate on each statement, and then personalise it in the spaces provided. You can also write your own affirmations. Remember, keep them positive and focus on what you want, rather than on what you don't want. Write and say them in the present tense.

I can communicate with my baby
at all times

*My cervix
knows how to open fully*

My baby descends naturally

Birthing is a time of pleasure

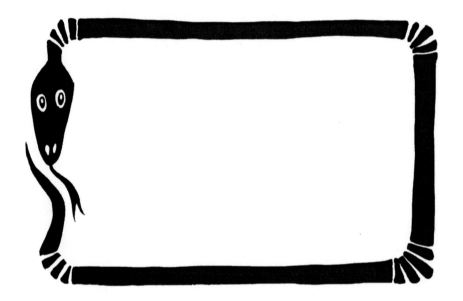

There is nothing to be feared

*The movements of my uterus
hug and massage my baby
during birthing*

The Birthkeepers

I enjoy birthing my baby

My birthing affirmations

My birthing plan

This is where I'd like to give birth:

This is what is important to me during birth:

This is what I will do to create the birth of my dreams:

These are the sights, smells, sounds and comforts that I would like around me at birth:

It is my baby's birthright to be born gently, peacefully and beautifully. This is what I will believe in order to help this happen:

About the artist:

Andri Thwaites is passionate about horticulture and garden design. Her art includes: sculptural work in gardens; pottery; ceramic and textile murals; kids' workshops; and freelance illustrative work for The Mother magazine.

She lives with her husband, Tom, and their two children, Joe Bob and Silvi, on a permaculture-inspired farm in Cumbria.

Andri provided the cartoons for Veronika's book, The Drinks Are On Me ~ everything your mother never told you about breastfeeding.

About the author:

Veronika Sophia Robinson was born and raised in South East Queensland, Australia, the fourth of eight children. She now lives in the north of England, with her husband, Paul, and their two home-educated daughters, Bethany and Eliza.

Living at the base of the Pennines, Veronika derives inspiration and nourishment from her rural lifestyle.

She co-founded the National Waterbirth Trust (New Zealand) in 1995, and launched The Mother magazine to an international readership in 2002. Alongside editing this unique publication on optimal parenting, Veronika's other passions include being a wife and mother, metaphysics, psychological astrology, organic gardening, living in accord with Nature, self-sufficiency and music.

About the publisher:

Starflower Press is dedicated to publishing material which lifts the heart, and helps to raise human consciousness to a new level of awareness.

Starflower Press draws its name and inspiration from the olden day herb, Borage (Borago Officinalis), commonly known as Starflower. It is still found in many places, though it is often thought of as a wild flower, rather than a herb.

Starflower is recognisable by its beautiful star-like flowers, which are formed by five petals of intense blue (sometimes it is pink). The unusual blue colour was used in Renaissance paintings. The Biblical meaning of this blue is heavenly grace.

Borage, from the Celt borrach, means courage. Throughout history, Starflower has been associated with courage. It is used as a food, tea, tincture and flower essence to bring joy to the heart and gladden the mind.

Visit www.starflowerpress.com for books, Starflower tea and Starflower Essence.

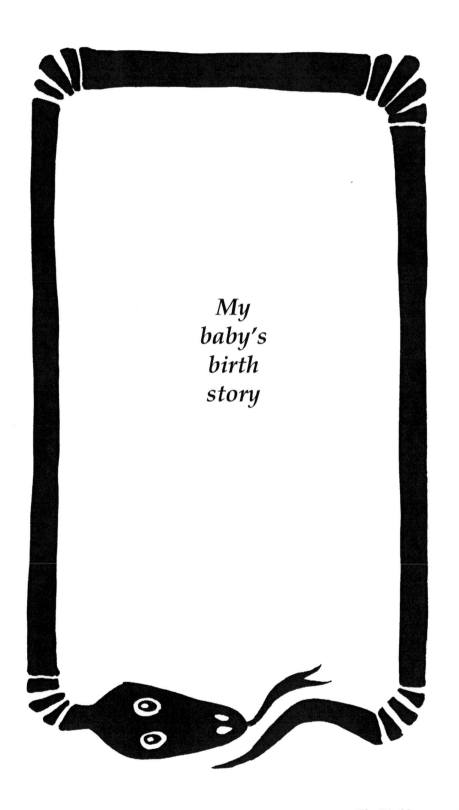

My baby's birth story

CPSIA information can be obtained at www.ICGtesting.com
Printed in the USA
BVOW02s0353210716

456299BV00016B/134/P